MAYO CLINIC ON
HIGH BLOOD PRESSURE

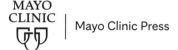
MAYO CLINIC | Mayo Clinic Press

MAYO CLINIC PRESS

Medical Editor Gary L. Schwartz, M.D.
Publisher Daniel J. Harke
Editor in Chief Nina E. Wiener
Managing Editor Stephanie K. Vaughan
Art Director Stewart J. Koski
Illustration and Photography Mayo Clinic Media Support Services, Mayo Clinic Medical Illustration and Animation
Editorial Research Librarian Anthony J. Cook
Contributors Brent A. Bauer, M.D.; Robert D. Brown Jr., M.D., M.P.H.; Matthew A. Clark, Ph.D., L.P.; Erin M. Dahlen, R.N.; Vesna D. Garovic, M.D., Ph.D.; James R. Gregoire, M.D.; J. Taylor Hays, M.D.; Stephen Kopecky, M.D.; Carrie A. Krieger, Pharm.D., R.Ph.; Edward R. Laskowski, M.D.; Francisco Lopez-Jimenez, M.D., M.B.A.; Sandra J. Taler, M.D.; Katherine A. Zeratsky, RDN, LD

Additional contributions from Kirkus Reviews and Rath Indexing

Image Credits All photographs and illustrations are copyright of Mayo Foundation for Medical Education and Research (MFMER) except for the following: NAME: 1296887873/COVER/CREDIT: © iStock/Getty Images Plus − NAME: GettyImages-1420728939/CHAPTER 2/ page 34/CREDIT: © GettyImages − NAME: 152961785-WomanTakingModernBP/CHAPTER 10/page 164/ CREDIT: © THINKSTOCK − NAME: 454113285-Take-ModernBP/CHAPTER 10/page 165/CREDIT: © THINKSTOCK

When you purchase Mayo Clinic newsletters and books, proceeds are used to further medical education and research at Mayo Clinic. You not only get answers to your questions on health, you become part of the solution.

Published by Mayo Clinic Press

© 2023 Mayo Foundation for Medical Education and Research (MFMER)

This book is adapted from *Mayo Clinic 5 Steps to Controlling High Blood Pressure*.

MAYO, MAYO CLINIC and the Mayo triple-shield logo are marks of Mayo Foundation for Medical Education and Research. All rights reserved. No part of this book may be reproduced, stored in a retrieval system, or transmitted, in any form or by any means, electronic, mechanical, photocopying, recording or otherwise, without the prior written permission of the publisher.

The information in this book is true and complete to the best of our knowledge. This book is intended only as an informative guide for those wishing to learn more about health issues. It is not intended to replace, countermand or conflict with advice given to you by your own physician. The ultimate decision concerning your care should be made between you and your doctor. Information in this book is offered with no guarantees. The author and publisher disclaim all liability in connection with the use of this book.

For bulk sales to employers, member groups and health-related companies, contact Mayo Clinic, 200 First St. SW, Rochester, MN 55905, or send an email to SpecialSalesMayoBooks@mayo.edu.

To stay informed about Mayo Clinic Press, please subscribe to our free e-newsletter at MCPress.MayoClinic.org or follow us on social media.

ISBN 9781945564758 (paperback)
9781945564109 (hardcover)
Library of Congress Control Number: 2022942481

Printed in China

Table of Contents

Preface

Blood pressure is the driving force that gets oxygen-rich blood — the body's life source — to your organs and tissues and delivers waste to your lungs, liver and kidneys for removal. With the right amount of pressure, the proper amount of blood travels throughout the body.

But when blood pressure is too high, blood flow to organs and tissues also becomes too high. In response, the muscular walls in the blood vessels narrow. This action restores balance in your blood flow, which is good, but the longer the blood vessels do this, the more stress they experience. Over time, the walls of the blood vessels thicken. This makes it hard to achieve proper blood flow, and blood pressure rises even more. In time, the increased stress on the blood vessels leads to organ damage.

This is the cycle of high blood pressure — and why it's so important to treat and prevent it.

While blood pressure naturally rises with age, it's not guaranteed that you'll develop high blood pressure — even if it runs in your family. And if you have high blood pressure already, you're far from doomed. You can control your destiny, helping your body find its right balance and lowering your blood pressure.

This book offers a solid understanding of the ways you can control your blood pressure — and your future. Taking the steps outlined in this book will help you reach a healthy blood pressure level and live well for years to come.

Gary L. Schwartz, M.D.

Gary L. Schwartz, M.D., is the head of the hypertension section within the Division of Nephrology and Hypertension in the Department of Internal Medicine at Mayo Clinic in Rochester, Minn. In his 40-plus years of studying, researching and treating people with high blood pressure, Dr. Schwartz has authored and reviewed numerous scientific papers and book chapters and has lectured around the world on topics related to blood pressure.

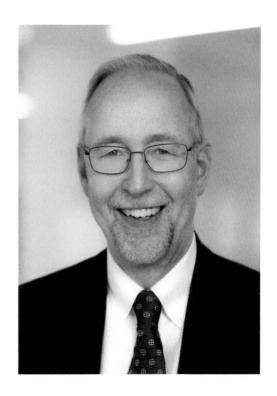

How high blood pressure develops

1

To understand how high blood pressure develops, it's useful to start with the basics about how the cardiovascular system and the organs that help regulate it work.

Each beat of the heart releases a surge of nutrient- and oxygen-rich blood from the heart's main pumping chamber (left ventricle) into a network of blood vessels (see "Cardiovascular system" illustration on page 11). The arteries are the blood vessels that carry blood from your heart to the rest of the body. The largest artery, called the aorta, is connected to the left ventricle. It serves as the main channel from the heart. The aorta branches into smaller arteries, which branch into even smaller arteries called arterioles. These tiny arteries narrow and widen to regulate the amount of blood that goes to an organ or tissue.

Tiny vessels called capillaries carry blood from the arterioles into the body's tissues. Capillaries are the final pathways for blood to get to the tissues inside the organs. Capillaries exchange nutrients and fresh oxygen for carbon dioxide and other waste products produced by the body's cells. Oxygen-depleted blood then returns to the heart through a system of blood vessels called veins.

When the blood in the veins reaches the heart, it's routed to the lungs, where it releases carbon dioxide and picks up a new supply of oxygen. With a fresh supply of oxygen, the blood is sent back to the

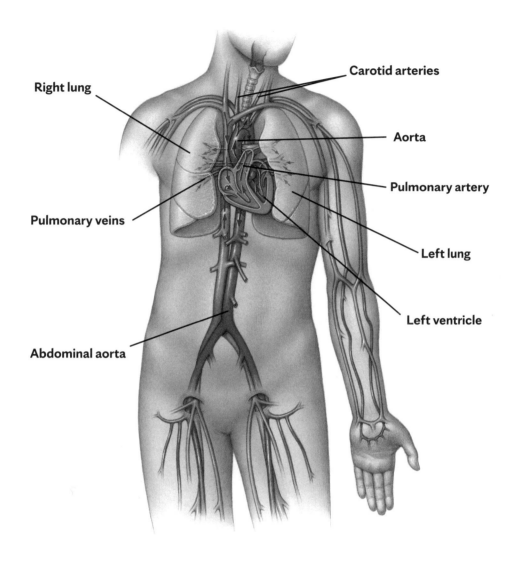

Each time the heart beats, blood is pumped from the left side of the heart (left ventricle) into the large blood vessel (aorta) that transports blood to the arteries (in red). As blood is pumped into the aorta, the aorta expands and holds on to some of the blood, which is then delivered to the arteries between heartbeats. This is how blood flows continuously through the body. Blood returns to the heart through the veins (in blue). Before being recirculated, the blood is sent to the lungs through the pulmonary artery to release waste products and load up on fresh oxygen.

heart, ready to resume the journey through the cardiovascular system. Other waste products are removed as blood passes through the kidneys and liver.

A certain amount of pressure — blood pressure — maintains this circulation and keeps all 11 pints of blood moving through the body at a rate that ensures the body gets the nutrients it needs and removes waste as needed. Blood pressure is the amount of force exerted on the artery walls to keep blood flowing.

Blood pressure is often compared to the pressure inside a garden hose. Without an exerting force, the water can't get from one end of the hose to the other.

REGULATORS OF BLOOD PRESSURE

Working together, several organs and body chemicals help control blood pressure. Together, this delicate system keeps blood pressure from rising too much or dropping too low and ensures that the body removes waste and gets the nutrients it needs. Even as blood pressure rises and falls throughout the day, these parts of the body keep tabs on these changes to ensure a healthy blood pressure level. Here's a look at each part of the system.

The heart

The flow of blood in the body starts with the heart. When blood leaves the heart from the left ventricle and moves into the aorta, a certain amount of force is created by the pumping action of the heart muscle. How fast and how strongly the heart beats influence the level of blood pressure. If the heart beats faster and more vigorously, blood pressure goes up. If it beats more slowly and less vigorously, blood pressure goes down.

Blood vessels

To accommodate the surge of blood coming from the heart, the arteries are lined with smooth muscles that allow the vessels to expand and contract as blood courses through them. If the blood vessels narrow (constrict), blood pressure goes up. If they widen (dilate), blood pressure tends to go down.

The walls of the blood vessels are lined with an extremely thin layer of cells called the endothelium. This tissue layer secretes chemicals that cause the blood vessels to relax or contract. For example, the endothelium contains nitric oxide that, when released, tells the smooth muscles in blood vessel walls to relax and expand, increasing blood flow and lowering pressure.

The endothelium also releases a protein called endothelin, which causes blood vessels to become narrow. Narrowed blood vessels reduce blood flow and raise blood pressure.

Adrenal glands

The adrenal glands, located above each kidney, produce three of the most

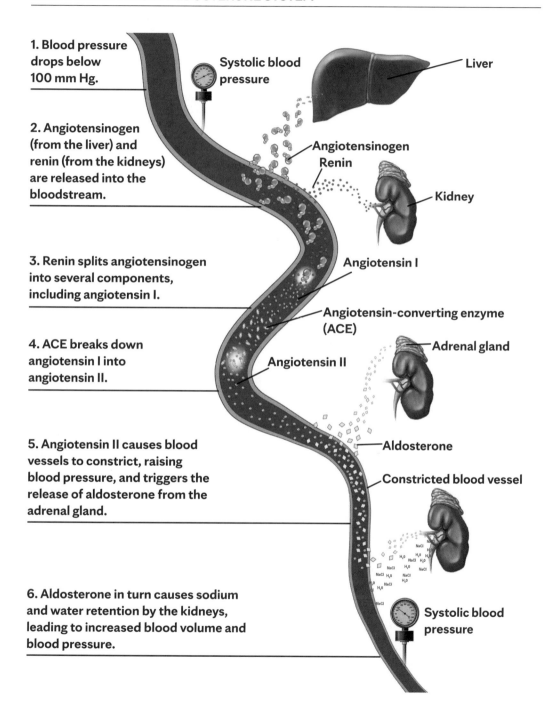

1. Blood pressure drops below 100 mm Hg.

Systolic blood pressure

Liver

2. Angiotensinogen (from the liver) and renin (from the kidneys) are released into the bloodstream.

Angiotensinogen
Renin

Kidney

3. Renin splits angiotensinogen into several components, including angiotensin I.

Angiotensin I

Angiotensin-converting enzyme (ACE)

4. ACE breaks down angiotensin I into angiotensin II.

Adrenal gland

Angiotensin II

5. Angiotensin II causes blood vessels to constrict, raising blood pressure, and triggers the release of aldosterone from the adrenal gland.

Aldosterone

Constricted blood vessel

NaCl
H₂O
NaCl

6. Aldosterone in turn causes sodium and water retention by the kidneys, leading to increased blood volume and blood pressure.

Systolic blood pressure

important hormones that affect blood pressure. Two of these are epinephrine, also known as adrenaline, and norepinephrine.

These hormones cause the arteries to narrow and the heart to pump harder and more rapidly. People often refer to the effect of the release of these hormones as feeling pumped up or being on an adrenaline high. Epinephrine and norepinephrine are released from the adrenal glands during periods of high stress or tension, such as when you're scared, in an argument or in a hurry. Epinephrine and norepinephrine are often called fight-or-flight hormones.

The adrenal glands also release aldosterone. This hormone causes the kidneys to retain sodium and water and excrete potassium.

The effects of these hormones and neurotransmitters help the body make short-term adjustments to blood pressure. In some people, the level of these hormones and neurotransmitters is higher than necessary, causing the blood pressure to be chronically higher. In turn, the higher blood pressure leads to a gradual thickening of the heart muscle and blood vessel walls, leading to impaired function and tissue damage.

The kidneys

An important role of the kidneys is to balance the amount of sodium and water in the body. Too much sodium and water raises blood pressure. Too little lowers blood pressure. The kidneys also produce renin, which can raise blood pressure by triggering a cascade of events, which you'll learn about next.

The renin-angiotensin-aldosterone system

Renin works on the angiotensinogen protein, which triggers a complex process. During this process, the substance angiotensin II is formed. This substance narrows the blood vessels. When blood vessels narrow, blood pressure increases. See how this process works on page 13.

Angiotensin II also stimulates release of the hormone aldosterone. Increased levels of aldosterone cause the kidneys to retain more sodium and water, also increasing pressure.

How everything works together

The brain has a blood pressure control center. It receives many signals related to physical factors such as diet, exercise, obesity and stress. In turn, the blood pressure control center in the brain sends signals to all the regulators of blood pressure in the body, signaling them to adjust blood pressure to meet the changing needs of the body during daily life.

The blood pressure control center sends the signals it receives through a part of the nervous system called the autonomic nervous system. It's made up of two parts, the sympathetic nervous system and the parasympathetic nervous system.

Signals sent through the sympathetic nervous system increase blood pressure during stress-related activities. Signals sent through the parasympathetic nervous system return blood pressure to normal. Here's an example of how this system works: During exercise, blood pressure must increase so muscles get extra oxygen and nutrients. After exercise, blood pressure should lower when the muscles no longer need increased nutrients and oxygen.

In addition, within the walls of the heart and certain blood vessels are special cells called baroreceptors. Located near the arteries in the heart and neck, these cells provide important signals to the blood pressure control center. Just as a thermostat regulates the temperature of a house, baroreceptors monitor blood pressure.

If baroreceptors sense a pressure change, they send signals through the nerves to the blood pressure control center, telling it to adjust blood pressure to keep it in its usual range. However, the range used by the baroreceptors varies and can be reset in response to short-term changes in blood pressure, such as during exercise.

In short, a complicated system in the body makes sure that blood pressure rises and lowers as needed to keep average blood pressure within a safe range.

WHEN BLOOD PRESSURE IS PERSISTENTLY HIGH

When the complex system that regulates blood pressure doesn't work as it's supposed to, too much pressure may build up within the arteries. As a result, the arteries narrow to keep blood flowing at the proper rate. Over time, the stress that this process puts on the arteries causes them to thicken, making it harder for blood to flow through them. This leads to higher blood pressure. When this increased pressure is constant, you may be told that you have high blood pressure. Hypertension is the medical term for this condition.

Hypertension isn't the same as nervous tension. You can be a generally calm, relaxed person and still have high blood pressure.

It's also important to note that a high number in either diastolic or systolic blood pressure is harmful. For adults younger than 50, a high diastolic pressure is usually the main issue. For adults older than age 50, high systolic pressure tends to be more common. This is because diastolic blood pressure rises until midlife and then stays at that level before dropping later in life. Systolic blood pressure, on the other hand, rises throughout life.

High blood pressure usually develops slowly. Most often, blood pressure increases over time and eventually progresses to hypertension.

THE TOLL OF HIGH BLOOD PRESSURE

Left untreated, high blood pressure can damage many of the body's organs and tissues. The higher the blood pressure

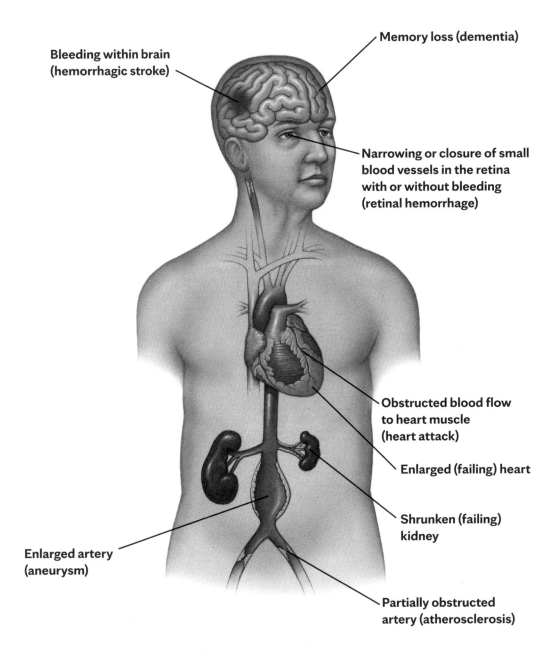

Bleeding within brain (hemorrhagic stroke)

Memory loss (dementia)

Narrowing or closure of small blood vessels in the retina with or without bleeding (retinal hemorrhage)

Obstructed blood flow to heart muscle (heart attack)

Enlarged (failing) heart

Shrunken (failing) kidney

Enlarged artery (aneurysm)

Partially obstructed artery (atherosclerosis)

Left untreated, high blood pressure can damage tissues and organs throughout the body. Sites in the body most affected by high blood pressure include the arteries, heart, brain, kidneys and eyes.

and the longer it goes untreated, the greater the risk that it will cause damage. When high blood pressure is combined with other factors or conditions, such as diabetes, obesity or tobacco use, the risk of injury from high blood pressure increases.

Plus, when high blood pressure is left untreated, it continues to rise over time and requires more treatment to lower and control it. The longer you wait to treat high blood pressure, the more damage that can be done. And if you wait too long to treat it, you may miss out on some of the benefits that medication can offer, as some damage can't be reversed when blood pressure has been too high for too long.

The parts of the body typically affected by high blood pressure include the arteries, heart, brain, kidneys and eyes (see illustration on page 16). Here's more on how high blood pressure affects each of these parts of the body.

The arteries

Persistent high blood pressure creates a heavier workload for the heart and the network of arteries that carry blood throughout the body. Read on to learn about the complications it can cause.

Arteriosclerosis

Healthy arteries are flexible, strong and elastic. Their inside lining is smooth so blood can flow through them unrestrict-ed. Too much pressure in the arteries over many years can make the walls thick, stiff and less elastic. This makes it hard for blood to flow. The medical term for this is arteriosclerosis, which comes from the Greek word sklerosis, meaning "hardening."

Atherosclerosis

High blood pressure speeds the buildup of fatty deposits in the arteries. Ather in the term atherosclerosis comes from the Greek word for "porridge," because the fatty deposits have the consistency of porridge. Many things can help lead to atherosclerosis, including smoking, high cholesterol, diabetes, inactivity and poor diet. If you have any of these risk factors for atherosclerosis, high blood pressure causes these deposits to develop more quickly.

When the inner wall of an artery is damaged, blood cells and fat cells often clump together at the injury site. They invade and scar deeper layers of the artery walls. Large accumulations of these fatty deposits are called plaques.

Over time, the plaques harden. The greatest danger of having plaques on blood vessel walls is that organs and tissues served by these narrowed arteries don't get enough blood, leading to blood vessel and organ scarring or symptoms from low blood flow. In turn, the heart increases pressure by pumping harder to maintain adequate blood flow. Increased pressure leads to further blood vessel damage.

Plaques also can cause other problems. As blood flows past the blockage, plaques may cause blood clots to form. In addition, inflammation often occurs in areas around plaques. Sometimes, plaques break apart and the pieces combine with fresh blood clots to block the artery. Debris may also travel in the bloodstream and lodge in a smaller artery.

ATHEROSCLEROSIS

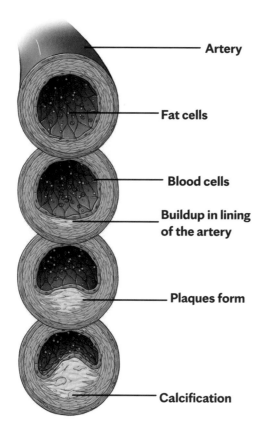

Artery

Fat cells

Blood cells

Buildup in lining of the artery

Plaques form

Calcification

The buildup of fatty deposits in the arteries leads to the formation of plaques, which can obstruct or block blood flow.

Arteriosclerosis and atherosclerosis can happen anywhere in the body but most often affect arteries in the heart, legs, neck, brain, kidneys and the major blood vessel that supplies blood to the body (abdominal aorta).

Aneurysm

When a blood vessel is damaged, part of the wall may bulge outward. This bulge is called an aneurysm. An aneurysm most commonly occurs in a brain artery or abdominal aorta (see page 19). If the aneurysm leaks or bursts, it can cause life-threatening internal bleeding.

Many brain aneurysms, particularly small ones, don't produce any signs or symptoms. But an aneurysm in a brain artery can sometimes lead to a sudden, extremely severe headache that's unlike any headache you've ever experienced. This headache is caused by bleeding surrounding the brain. A large abdominal aortic aneurysm may cause constant pain in the belly or lower back. Occasionally, a blood clot lining the aneurysm wall breaks off and obstructs an artery downstream.

Hypertension is a risk factor for aneurysms and a leading cause of brain aneurysms rupturing.

The heart

High blood pressure can put stress on the heart and keep it from working well. Here's more on the issues high blood pressure can cause for the heart.

Coronary artery disease

The buildup of plaques in the major arteries serving the heart is called coronary artery disease. It's common in people who have high blood pressure.

A temporary drop in blood supply to the heart causes chest pain, also known as angina. If the heart muscle is too deprived of blood, a heart attack may occur. This is when lack of blood flow causes the heart to stop working. The complications of coronary artery disease are the major causes of death in people with uncontrolled high blood pressure.

Reduced blood flow in the coronary arteries calls for an immediate trip to the emergency room and treatment with medication or a procedure for opening blood vessels (angioplasty) to prevent or limit permanent damage to heart muscle.

Left ventricular hypertrophy

When the heart pumps blood into the aorta, it pushes blood out against the resistance to flow that has built up in the arteries. Higher resistance causes higher pressure. The higher the pressure, the harder the heart must work and the larger the heart gets.

Eventually, the wall of the heart's main pumping chamber starts to thicken (hypertrophy) from the excessive workload. The enlarged left ventricle needs more blood. Because high blood pressure also causes the blood vessels feeding the heart to narrow, there's often not enough

blood going to the heart. Controlling high blood pressure can prevent this.

Heart failure

Heart failure occurs when the heart doesn't pump effectively and can't circulate enough blood to meet the body's needs. As a result, fluid backs up and

ANEURYSM

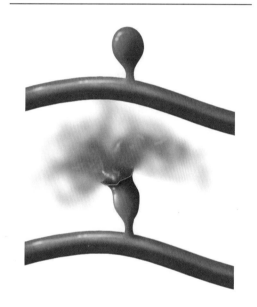

An aneurysm is a bulge or ballooning in the wall of a blood vessel. An aneurysm can burst (rupture), causing internal bleeding and often leading to death. Aneurysms usually don't cause symptoms, so you might not know you have an aneurysm even if it's large. An aneurysm most commonly occurs in a brain artery or in the lower part of the major vessel that supplies blood to the body (aorta).

builds up in the lungs, legs and other tissues, a condition called edema.

Fluid in the lungs leads to shortness of breath; fluid buildup in the legs causes swelling. By controlling high blood pressure, you can help reduce your risk of heart failure.

The brain

High blood pressure is the leading cause of stroke. A stroke is a type of brain injury caused by blocked or ruptured blood vessels that disrupt the brain's blood supply. Deprived of nutrients, brain cells are damaged or die. High blood pressure increases your risk of having a stroke. The lifetime risk of stroke for adults at age 55 with normal blood pressure is 1 in 5 for women and 1 in 6 for men. In people who have hypertension, the risk of stroke almost doubles.

There are two basic types of strokes. They differ based on the type of disturbance in the blood supply and location.

Ischemic strokes

Ischemic strokes are the most common type, accounting for nearly 90% of all strokes. They usually affect the part of the brain called the cerebrum, which controls movement, language and the senses.

An ischemic stroke may result from a blood clot that formed as a result of blockage from plaques. This type of stroke occurs if an artery that supplies oxygen-rich blood to the brain becomes blocked.

An ischemic stroke may also occur if a small piece of clotted blood breaks loose and is swept through larger arteries into smaller arteries in the brain. The moving (embolic) clot may get lodged and block blood flow, resulting in a stroke. Clot-busting drugs given within the first few hours after an ischemic stroke begins can greatly reduce disability from the stroke.

Sometimes the blockage may be removed from the artery using what's called an endovascular procedure. A small plastic tube called a catheter is inserted into an artery in the upper part of the leg and sent up into the brain artery. Through the tip of the catheter, a small device can then be sent into the blockage in the brain artery, and the blockage can sometimes be removed. This allows the blood flow to provide oxygen and other nutrients to the brain and may lessen the severity of the stroke.

Sometimes blood supply to the brain is briefly disrupted, for less than 24 hours. This is known as a transient ischemic attack (TIA). Its symptoms are like those of a stroke, but a TIA usually lasts only a few minutes or hours. It's important not to ignore these symptoms even if they go away. A TIA may be a warning — about 1 in 3 people who have a TIA will eventually have a stroke. Many of those strokes can be prevented with medical care immediately after the TIA and by taking steps toward preventing a stroke in the future.

Hemorrhagic strokes

A hemorrhagic stroke occurs when a blood vessel in the brain leaks or ruptures. The most common cause is high blood pressure; it causes a weakening in the artery wall, which can then sometimes rupture. A hemorrhage may also be caused by the development of a bulge in the blood vessel wall (aneurysm). Blood from the hemorrhage damages the surrounding brain tissue. In addition, tissue over a broader area is damaged because it's deprived of blood. High blood pressure can increase your risk of having a hemorrhagic stroke because it damages the arteries and can increase the risk of an aneurysm.

Improved detection and treatment of high blood pressure have led to a dramatic reduction in the number of strokes. When treatment lowers blood pressure, the risk of stroke decreases remarkably.

Even if you've had a stroke or TIA, lowering your blood pressure can help prevent these problems from recurring.

Treating, preventing stroke

If you think you or someone else may be having a stroke, think FAST:

Face. Ask the person to smile. Does one side of the face droop?
Arms. Ask the person to raise both arms. Does one arm drift downward? Or is one arm unable to rise?
Speech. Ask the person to repeat a simple phrase. Is speech slurred or strange?

Time. If you observe any of these signs, call 911 or emergency medical help immediately.

Note when the following signs and symptoms begin; the length of time they have been present may guide your treatment decisions.

Drugs injected into your veins or arteries can dissolve a blood clot — a common cause of stroke — when they're given

ISCHEMIC STROKE

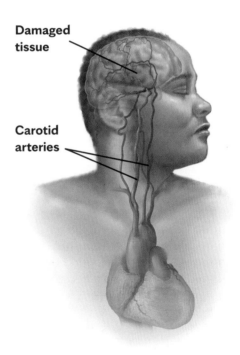

Damaged tissue

Carotid arteries

When blood flow in an artery leading to the brain is obstructed, nerve cells are deprived of oxygen and nutrients. Brain tissue quickly may be damaged or die.

within a few hours after the symptoms start. Sometimes the blockage is removed from the artery.

If you've had a stroke or TIA, your doctor may have you take a diuretic and an angiotensin-converting enzyme (ACE) inhibitor to help reduce your risk of a second stroke. Angiotensin II receptor blockers (ARBs) and calcium channel blockers also may be prescribed. Using these drugs to lower blood pressure can reduce the risk of another stroke even if you've never had high blood pressure. Research shows that diuretics or the combination of diuretics and an ACE inhibitor is useful in reducing stroke risk.

Aspirin and other drugs that inhibit blood clotting are important in preventing another stroke. In some cases, angioplasty and stenting or other surgical procedures on the carotid or other arteries, which provide blood flow to the brain, may be performed.

Dementia

High blood pressure can cause extensive narrowing and blockage of the small and large arteries that supply blood to the brain. If you already have a narrowing or blockage of these arteries, high blood pressure can make it worse. The reduced blood supply can lead to a series of small or even large strokes, leaving behind areas of damaged brain tissue.

Studies suggest that damaged blood vessels in the brain caused by high blood pressure can sometimes lead to dementia, a progressive brain disorder that often includes memory loss, disorientation and personality change.

As you age, the risk of Alzheimer's disease, dementia caused by small strokes (vascular dementia) and other types of dementia greatly increases. After a diagnosis of high blood pressure, dementia can appear anywhere from a few years to as many as several decades later. Recent evidence suggests that controlling high blood pressure with the help of medication may reduce the risk of dementia. Although existing damage to brain tissue can't be reversed, additional damage can be prevented.

The eyes

Occasionally, a simple eye exam leads to a diagnosis of hypertension because the small blood vessels of the retina often reflect the earliest and clearest indicators of high blood pressure.

In early stages, the tiny retinal arteries narrow. Eventually, the walls of the arteries thicken, pressing against nearby veins and making it hard for blood to flow through them. Retinal blood vessels may leak blood and fluid into the retinal tissue (see image on page 24).

In severe cases of high blood pressure, fluid may also leak into the optic nerve, which causes swelling in the nerve (papilledema). Severe hemorrhaging in the retina and optic nerve leads to vision loss. Controlling high blood pressure almost always prevents these complications.

The kidneys

When blood circulates through the kidneys, these organs filter out waste products and regulate the balance of minerals, acids and fluids in blood. Each kidney has over 1 million nephrons, tiny filtering systems made up of small blood vessels and attached tubes.

The kidneys help control blood pressure by regulating levels of sodium and water. They also produce angiotensin II, which, as you learned earlier, controls blood vessel size. High blood pressure can interfere with these functions. Atherosclerosis due to high blood pressure can reduce blood flow to the kidneys, preventing them from eliminating enough waste from the bloodstream. The waste builds up and the kidneys may stop functioning, leading to kidney failure.

If your kidneys stop functioning, you'll need to undergo kidney dialysis, a process by which the waste products in blood are filtered out by machine, or you may need a kidney transplant.

Damage without symptoms

If you have hypertension, it's likely you don't know it, without getting an accurate

HOW THE KIDNEYS WORK

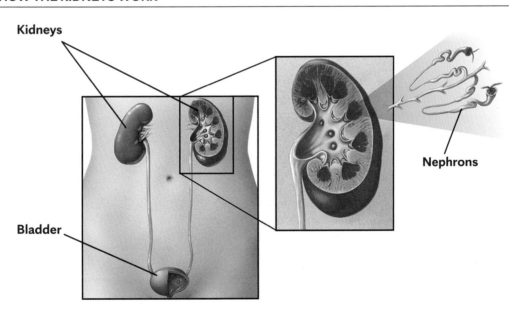

Kidneys

Nephrons

Bladder

Waste filtered from the blood by the kidneys is stored in the bladder as urine. Each kidney has more than a million nephrons that filter waste from the blood.

blood pressure reading. All the damage you've read about to this point happens without you even knowing that it's taking place. This is why hypertension is called a silent killer.

Some people think headaches, dizziness or nosebleeds are indications of high blood pressure. Although a few people may experience some nosebleeds or dizziness when their blood pressure rises, research has found no direct link between headaches and hypertension.

You can have high blood pressure for years without ever knowing it. The condition is most often discovered during routine physical exams. Symptoms such as shortness of breath typically don't occur until high blood pressure has advanced to an extremely high — possibly life-threatening — stage. And even

with very high blood pressure, some people experience no signs or symptoms until it has caused organ damage or reached an extremely high level.

MEASURING BLOOD PRESSURE

To determine the blood pressure in your arteries — and whether you have high blood pressure — a member of your health care team will use an instrument called a sphygmomanometer. This device includes an inflatable cuff that's wrapped around your upper arm, an air pump and a digital meter. When the cuff is inflated it squeezes the blood vessels in the arm.

Today, most devices are automated. They determine blood pressure by sensing the movement of the arterial wall beneath the cuff as the cuff is inflated or deflated.

DAMAGE TO THE RETINA

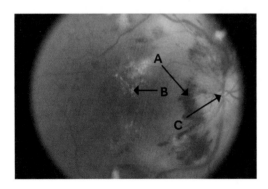
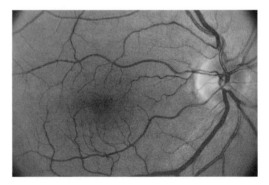

Shown on the left, blood vessels in the retina may rupture (A) because of high blood pressure, causing bleeding (hemorrhaging) and a buildup (B) of waste deposits (exudates). Tissue swelling as a result of a combination of leakage and inflammation (C) may include the optic nerve (papilledema). The image of a healthy retina is shown on the right.

Blood pressure is expressed in terms of millimeters of mercury (mm Hg). The measurement refers to how high the pressure in the arteries can raise a column of mercury in the pressure gauge on a sphygmomanometer.

You'll likely have two or more blood pressure readings taken at three or more separate appointments before being diagnosed with high blood pressure. For each measurement, you should be in a seated position.

You may have blood pressure measured in both arms to determine if there's a difference between the two. The arm with the higher blood pressure is the one that will likely be used to measure your blood pressure going forward.

Two numbers are included in a blood pressure reading. They're often written to look like a fraction.

The top number is called systolic pressure. This is the amount of pressure the

PUMPING ACTION OF THE HEART

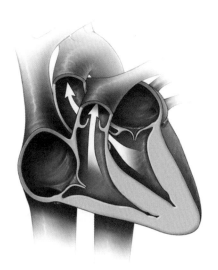

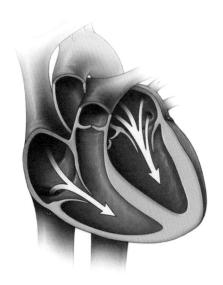

Systole (pumping)　　　　　　**Diastole (resting)**

During systole (left), the heart muscle squeezes blood out of the heart's pumping chambers (ventricles). Blood on the right side of the heart goes to the lungs, and blood on the left side is pumped into the large blood vessel (aorta) that feeds the arteries. During diastole (right), the heart muscle relaxes and expands to allow blood to flow into the pumping chambers from the heart's holding chambers (atria).

heart produces when it pumps blood through the arteries to the rest of the body.

The bottom number is called diastolic pressure. This is the amount of pressure that stays in the arteries when the heart is at rest between beats. The heart muscle must relax fully before it contracts again. Blood pressure decreases until the next contraction.

When stated verbally, the word "over" is used to separate the two numbers. For example, if your systolic pressure is 115 mm Hg and your diastolic pressure is 82 mm Hg, your blood pressure is written as 115/82, and spoken as "115 over 82."

WHAT'S TOO HIGH?

For adults, blood pressure below 120/80 mm Hg is the level at which it poses no negative health consequences or risks for most people. This is often described as normal blood pressure.

Blood pressure is described as elevated when systolic blood pressure (the top

BLOOD PRESSURE CLASSIFICATIONS FOR ADULTS

	Systolic (mm Hg*) (top number)		Diastolic (mm Hg) (bottom number)
Normal	Less than 120	and	Less than 80
Elevated	120 to 129	and	Less than 80
Hypertension Stage 1[†] Stage 2[†]	130 to 139 140 or higher	or or	80 to 89 90 or higher
Hypertensive crisis	Higher than 180	and/or	Higher than 120

*Millimeters of mercury

[†]Based on the average of two or more readings taken in a seated position and taken on two or more visits. Systolic hypertension is a major risk factor for cardio-vascular disease, even without elevated diastolic pressure, especially in older people.

Source: Whelton PK, et al. 2017. Guideline for the Prevention, Detection, Evaluation, and Management of High Blood Pressure in Adults.

- Blood pressure is necessary to keep blood flowing through the heart and blood vessels.
- High blood pressure means you have high blood pressure readings on a persistent basis. That means systolic blood pressure is consistently 120 mm Hg or higher, diastolic pressure is consistently 80 mm Hg or higher, or both.
- High blood pressure typically doesn't produce any signs or symptoms.
- Left untreated, high blood pressure can lead to stroke, heart attack, heart and kidney failure, blindness and dementia.
- By controlling high blood pressure, you significantly reduce your risk of disability or death related to the disease.

number) is between 120 and 129 mm Hg and diastolic pressure (the bottom number) is less than 80 mm Hg. This means that your blood pressure is higher than it should be but isn't in the high blood pressure range. Having elevated blood pressure also means you have a higher risk of heart disease, kidney disease and stroke.

If you have elevated blood pressure, your blood pressure should be monitored regularly as you work to lower it. Elevated blood pressure tends to worsen over time if steps aren't taken to control it.

High blood pressure is diagnosed when blood pressure reaches 130/80 mm Hg and higher. Hypertension is diagnosed in two categories, stage 1 and stage 2, depending on your systolic and diastolic pressures.

USING KNOWLEDGE TO YOUR ADVANTAGE

With a base idea of what high blood pressure is and all the ways it can affect the body, you're on your way to taking steps toward lowering your blood pressure if it's high and keeping it in check if it's not. Later on, you'll learn the best steps to take to lower your blood pressure if it's high and keep it at a level that's healthy for you.

2

Who's at risk?

With any disease, you likely want to know its cause. Why does a condition occur in some people but not in others? Why does it develop in most adults after a certain age, but for some people, the symptoms appear 10 or 20 years earlier? With high blood pressure, the reasons why it occurs in most people are often unknown.

However, it's clear that certain factors can put you at greater risk of high blood pressure. By knowing what these factors are, you can take steps to lessen the risk and delay or even prevent high blood pressure from occurring.

To understand your risk, it's important to first know that there are two forms of high blood pressure: primary and secondary. Primary high blood pressure is also known as "essential" high blood pressure. The word "essential" is tied to a time when elevated blood pressure was considered a normal change the body made in response to reduced blood flow to organs and tissues. By that definition, this was considered an essential change; treatment to lower it was seen as harmful.

It's estimated that 90% to 95% of people with high blood pressure have essential high blood pressure. Essential high blood pressure has no obvious cause, but certain genetic traits and lifestyle habits — such as diet, lack of physical activity and being overweight — play important roles in its development.

In 5% to 10% of people with high blood pressure, a cause can be identified. This is called secondary high blood pressure. This means that high blood pressure is due to — or "secondary" to — another condition. Unlike the essential or primary form, secondary high blood pressure may be correctable. When the underlying condition is treated, blood pressure may decrease or even return to a healthy level, reducing the risk of complications.

Here's more on each of these two types of hypertension.

PRIMARY HIGH BLOOD PRESSURE

Among most Americans with high blood pressure, it's hard to pinpoint the exact cause. This is known as primary high blood pressure.

Genes may play an important role in the development of high blood pressure. But researchers are discovering that high blood pressure is a complex illness that doesn't typically follow the classic rules of genetic inheritance. Instead of stemming from a single defective gene, high blood pressure seems to be a multifaceted disorder that, except in rare cases, involves interaction among multiple or many genes, with any single gene having only a small effect on blood pressure.

Essential hypertension is the result of a complex interaction of genetic variation and environmental factors. Thirty percent of the variation in blood pressure among people is due to genetic differences, and 70% is due to environmental factors.

Although you can't change your genes (at least not yet), you can control the environmental factors that interact with your genes to produce high blood pressure. Environmental factors are considered risk factors for the development of hypertension.

Primary high blood pressure results from a combination of factors related to:
- Motion (widening and narrowing) of your blood vessels.
- Increased fluid in your blood.
- Functioning of your blood flow sensors (baroreceptors).
- Production of chemicals that influence blood vessel function.
- Secretion of hormones that affect your cardiovascular system.
- The volume of blood the heart pumps.
- Nerve control of your cardiovascular system.

Risk factors such as weight, sodium use, too little potassium in your diet and physical activity also appear to interact with genetic factors.

Generally, the more of these risk factors you have, the greater the odds that you'll have high blood pressure in your lifetime. That's because genetic and environmental interactions influence the many physiological factors that cause blood pressure to increase over time, as you learned in Chapter 1.

Risk factors you can't change

There are four major risk factors you can't change or control.

Race

About a third of white Americans age 18 and older have high blood pressure. Among Black Americans, the number jumps to 45%. High blood pressure affects a third of Mexican Americans and Asians.

Age

The risk of high blood pressure increases with age. Americans whose blood pressure is at a healthy level at age 55 still have a 90% lifetime risk of developing high blood pressure. Part of this risk is related to factors you can change, so paying attention to risk factors within your control can help you reduce the risk of developing hypertension.

Family history

A family history may reflect genetic factors that are inherited. However, it may also reflect environmental factors that are shared or learned in families. Hypertension develops as the result of the interaction of a genetic predisposition with the environment. Though you can't change your genes, you can change your environment.

Sex

Through about age 45, high blood pressure is more common in men. But after age 65, women are more likely than men to develop the condition.

Risk factors you can change

Though there are risk factors you can't control, there are many ways you can lower your risk of high blood pressure. Here's a brief look at each risk factor. At the end of this chapter, you'll get several ideas to help you make changes in these areas.

Weight

Being overweight increases your risk of high blood pressure for several reasons.

The greater your body mass, the more blood and blood vessels you need to nourish your cells. Since the heart pumps approximately 100,000 times a day, weight gain as an adult increases the workload of the healthy heart by increasing the miles of blood vessels in the body. More blood circulating through the arteries requires the heart to pump with greater force. Obesity is also associated with increased activity in the sympathetic nervous system and higher levels of aldosterone, both of which can raise blood pressure.

Excess weight can increase your heart rate. It also increases the level of insulin in your blood, causing your body to retain more sodium and water.

In addition, some people who are overweight follow a diet that's too high in saturated fat and trans fat. These fats promote atherosclerosis, which causes the arteries to narrow. Find guidance on how much fat to include in your diet in Chapter 5.

Diet

Diet plays a role in the risk of high blood pressure in a handful of ways that you can control.

Sodium

The body's cells need a certain amount of the essential mineral sodium to stay healthy. A common source of sodium is table salt (sodium chloride), which is composed of about 40% sodium and 60% chloride.

On average, the salt in processed foods makes up 70% of your sodium intake. Since there's no health-related reason to consume excess salt, almost everyone can benefit from reducing sodium intake. For more on sodium intake, see Chapter 5.

Potassium

Potassium is a mineral that helps balance the amount of sodium in the body's cells. It gets rid of excess sodium by way of the kidneys, which filter out the sodium that will be excreted in the urine. If you don't get enough potassium in your diet or your body can't retain a proper amount, too much sodium can build up, increasing the risk of high blood pressure. Potassium also helps blood vessels relax and helps blood flow more easily, which lowers blood pressure. Learn more about potassium in Chapter 5.

Caffeine

Caffeine may cause a short, but dramatic increase in your blood pressure. Though it's unclear what causes this spike, it

A CLOSER LOOK AT OBESITY

More than 4 in 10 adults are overweight, and that number is expected to jump to 1 in 2 by 2030.

But adults aren't the only ones putting on excess weight. Data from a worldwide analysis shows that nearly 1 in 5 children in developed countries — boys and girls alike — are overweight or obese. For children and adolescents in developing countries, the rate is also on the rise. Rates of high blood pressure are higher in children and adolescents who are overweight.

Excess weight is second only to smoking as a leading cause of preventable death in the United States. In 2000, about 365,000 U.S. deaths were associated with being overweight or obesity. In comparison, it's estimated that 480,000 deaths a year were associated with cigarette smoking.

could be that caffeine blocks a hormone that keeps the arteries widened. Or it may cause the adrenal glands to release more adrenaline, leading to an increase in blood pressure. Limiting intake to 200 milligrams a day — about two cups of coffee — can help.

Too little exercise

Lack of physical activity increases the risk of high blood pressure by making obesity more likely. People who are inactive also tend to have higher heart rates, and their heart has to work harder with each contraction. The harder and more often the heart has to pump, the greater the force exerted on the arteries.

Tobacco use

The chemicals in tobacco can damage the lining of the artery walls, making them more prone to the buildup of plaques. Nicotine increases heart rate and causes the blood vessels to narrow by triggering hormone production, which in turn raises blood pressure. These effects occur because tobacco use triggers hormone production, including increased levels of epinephrine (adrenaline).

In addition, carbon monoxide in cigarette smoke replaces oxygen in the blood. This can increase blood pressure by making the heart work harder to get enough oxygen to the body's cells. Smoking is the single most important risk factor for an aortic aneurysm, a bulging section in the wall of the aorta that may rupture or cause a blood clot to form. For details on stopping smoking, see Chapter 7.

Stress

If stress episodes occur often enough, they can damage blood vessels, heart and kidneys.

Although blood pressure may increase temporarily when you're under stress, stress has not been proven to cause chronic high blood pressure. However, recent research shows that people who have an anxiety disorder may be more likely to develop high blood pressure. Stress can also promote unhealthy habits that are known to increase the risk of hypertension. For example, some people turn to smoking, drinking alcohol or overeating to relieve stress. For more on stress and high blood pressure, see Chapter 10.

Metabolic syndrome

Metabolic syndrome involves all of the risk factors you've learned about so far. It's a cluster of modifiable conditions that occur together — including high blood pressure, elevated blood sugar, excess body weight, a low level of high-density lipoprotein (HDL, or "good") cholesterol, and a high level of triglycerides, a type of fat found in the blood. Together, these conditions make it more likely that you'll have diabetes, heart disease and a stroke.

If you have all or even some of the syndrome's risk factors, take steps to reduce your risk of life-threatening illnesses. For more on metabolic syndrome, see pages 144-145.

A multiplying effect

Risk factors usually don't exist independently of each other and often interact with each other. For example, if you're overweight and inactive, your odds of developing high blood pressure are much higher than if you have just one of these risk factors.

By the same token, working to reduce one risk factor may help you reduce other risk factors. For example, exercise and weight loss may improve diabetes and cholesterol and reduce risk of a heart attack or kidney disease in addition to reducing your risk of developing hypertension. Your total reduction in risk may be more than the sum of that one factor alone.

An important note to keep in mind: Although having risk factors affects your chances of developing high blood pressure, it's no guarantee of that happening. At the same time, it's possible to develop high blood pressure even if you have no risk factors.

Bottom line: Lessening or managing risk factors within your control reduces your odds of developing high blood pressure.

SECONDARY HIGH BLOOD PRESSURE

Secondary high blood pressure differs from primary high blood pressure because it's directly caused by another disorder. Secondary causes make up about 5% to 10% of the total cases of hypertension.

Secondary high blood pressure usually comes on more quickly than primary high blood pressure and pushes blood pressure to higher levels. When the underlying disease or condition is corrected, blood pressure typically decreases. In some people, blood pressure levels may return to normal.

Secondary hypertension can be caused by a variety of conditions. Here's more about each of these causes of high blood pressure.

First things first

Medications are a common cause of secondary high blood pressure, but alcohol and sleep apnea are often linked to hypertension, too.

Drugs and supplements

Several types of drugs can increase blood pressure in some people.

Many over-the-counter medications can have this effect include:
- Nonsteroidal anti-inflammatory drugs (NSAIDs) such as ibuprofen (Advil, Motrin IB, others) and naproxen sodium (Aleve)
- Appetite suppressants
- Cold remedies
- Nasal decongestants, including sprays

MEDICATIONS THAT LOWER BLOOD PRESSURE AS A SIDE EFFECT

Just as some medications can raise blood pressure, many medications can cause your blood pressure to drop and affect hypertension treatment. This is a partial list of medications that may cause a drop in blood pressure. Drugs are listed by the condition they are used to treat or by their drug type or class.

Alzheimer's disease drugs
- Donepezil (Aricept)
- Galantamine (Razadyne ER)

Antidepressants
- Trazodone
- Tricyclic antidepressants

Antiparkinsonian drugs
- Pramipexole (Mirapex ER)
- Ropinirole
- Carbidopa/levodopa (Sinemet)

Antipsychotics
- Olanzapine (Zyprexa)
- Quetiapine (Seroquel)
- Risperidone (Risperdal)

Narcotic analgesics
- Codeine
- Morphine

Erectile dysfunction (impotence, or ED) medications
- Sildenafil (Viagra, Revatio)
- Tadalafil (Cialis, Adcirca)
- Vardenafil (Levitra, Staxyn)

Antidiabetic drugs known as SGLT2 inhibitors
- Canagliflozin (Invokana)
- Dapagliflozin (Farxiga)
- Empagliflozin (Jardiance)

Several prescription medications can also affect blood pressure:

- Steroids (prednisolone, methylprednisolone)
- Antidepressants (bupropion; desipramine and other tricyclic antidepressants; phenelzine and other monoamine oxidase inhibitors; venlafaxine and desvenlafaxine; others)
- Immunosuppressants (cyclosporine, tacrolimus, others)
- COX-2 inhibitors (celecoxib)
- Others (epoetin alfa, also known as erythropoietin; darbepoetin alfa; methylphenidate and other stimulants; ergot alkaloids; some monoclonal antibodies, such as bevacizumab; and some kinase inhibitors, such as sorafenib and sunitinib)

Most birth control pills can increase blood pressure, but the effect may be less pronounced in birth control pills that have lower levels of progestin and estrogen. Drospirenone, a component of a contraceptive pill (Yasmin, Yaz, others), can cause the body to retain potassium and interfere with certain medications that are used to treat high blood pressure.

Certain products associated with complementary medicine can increase blood pressure or interfere with the effectiveness of blood pressure medications. These include bitter orange, ginseng, caffeinated energy drinks, licorice root, yohimbine and St. John's wort.

Street drugs, such as cocaine, can lead to high blood pressure by narrowing certain arteries, increasing heart rate or damaging the heart muscle.

Alcohol

Consuming three or more drinks of alcohol a day significantly raises the risk of high blood pressure. How or why alcohol increases blood pressure isn't fully understood. But over time, heavy drinking can damage the heart and other organs.

The safest course is to drink moderately or not at all. For most men, moderate drinking means no more than two alcoholic drinks a day. For women, the limit is one drink daily. One drink is equal to one 12-ounce bottle of beer, one 5-ounce glass of wine or one 1.5-ounce shot glass of 80-proof liquor.

Note that these are general recommendations for alcohol consumption, and individual guidelines may vary. For more on alcohol and high blood pressure, see Chapter 7.

Sleep apnea

Obstructive sleep apnea is a severe form of snoring that interrupts breathing during sleep. Interrupted sleep can also be due to a disturbance in brain function. Studies show a link between the interrupted breathing that happens during sleep apnea and the onset of high blood pressure.

Sleep apnea is common among people with high blood pressure, but experts aren't certain about how often sleep apnea causes high blood pressure. It is known, however, that sleep apnea increases the risk of stroke and heart rhythm issues such as atrial fibrillation.

If you consistently have trouble getting a restful night's sleep, awaken at night choking or gasping, and have trouble staying awake during the day, talk to your health care team. These can all be signs and symptoms of sleep apnea. Being overweight or obese also contributes to your risk.

Treatment may include losing weight, sleeping on your side rather than on your back and using a mask device that gently blows air through your airway with just enough pressure to keep the passage open.

Key causes of secondary high blood pressure

Chronic kidney disease, primary hyperaldosteronism and renal artery disease all increase the risk of developing secondary hypertension. Here's more on each condition and the effects they have on high blood pressure.

Kidney disease

Kidney disease is both a cause and an effect of chronic high blood pressure. The scarring of kidney tissue and narrowing of kidney blood vessels cause the kidneys to no longer get rid of sodium, water and waste products as they usually do. This leads to a buildup of salt and water in the body, which raises blood pressure. Damaged kidneys may also release

chemicals within the body that raise blood pressure (see pages 146-147). In the U.S., about 1 in 7 people has chronic kidney disease. There's a strong link between chronic kidney disease and hypertension.

Diabetes is one of many causes of kidney disease. When there's too much glucose in the blood, it can damage many organs and tissues, leading to conditions that cause high blood pressure, including kidney disease.

Kidney diseases such as polycystic kidney disease, glomerulonephritis and scleroderma can also cause damage that leads to kidney failure. Chronic kidney failure can progress to a point where either dialysis or a kidney transplant is the only treatment option available.

If it's possible that you have kidney disease, you'll have a physical exam. Tests that detect elevated levels of waste products in your blood and excess protein in your urine may indicate that your kidneys aren't working as they should. Imaging tests such as ultrasound, computerized tomography (CT) or magnetic resonance imaging (MRI) can reveal cysts or scars caused by kidney disease.

Primary hyperaldosteronism

Higher levels of aldosterone cause the kidneys to retain sodium and water, increasing blood pressure. Primary hyperaldosteronism is a common and potentially curable cause of secondary hypertension.

With primary hyperaldosteronism, the body produces too much aldosterone. Extra aldosterone is produced either by a tumor on one adrenal gland or when both glands grow in an unusual way.

As many as 1 in 10 adults has primary hyperaldosteronism. In addition, as many as 1 in 5 adults whose hypertension cannot be controlled despite multiple medications (resistant hypertension) has this condition.

Your health care team may suspect that you have this condition if your potassium level is low or if ordinary drug treatment doesn't lower your blood pressure. If it's possible you have this condition, you may have blood and urine tests and imaging with CT or MRI. Sampling of adrenal veins can help locate a tumor, particularly when it's too small to be seen using an imaging test. Treatment may include taking drugs or surgery to remove the adrenal gland that contains the tumor.

KIDNEY PROBLEMS

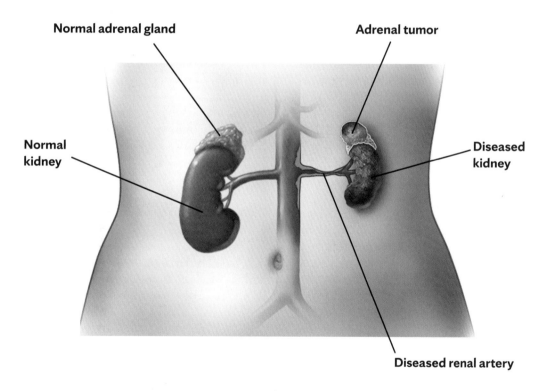

Normal adrenal gland

Adrenal tumor

Normal kidney

Diseased kidney

Diseased renal artery

Among common causes of secondary hypertension are narrowing of the renal artery and overproduction of a hormone from the adrenal gland (hyperaldosteronism).

Renal artery disease

The renal artery is the main vessel supplying blood to each kidney. Obstruction is often the result of a narrowing of the artery caused by atherosclerosis. When the obstruction is severe, the kidney may shrink and scar irreversibly. A narrowed renal artery due to atherosclerosis is the most common cause of secondary hypertension in people age 65 or older.

Obstruction can also be caused by a condition called fibromuscular dysplasia. In this condition, the middle layer of the artery wall (known as the media) thickens, narrowing the artery. The artery may have narrowed sections alternating with widened sections, which may form small aneurysms. One or both kidneys may be affected. This form of secondary hypertension is common in women in the child-bearing age range, but some don't learn they have the disorder until their later years.

Narrowing of the arteries can impair kidney function and lead to the production of the hormone renin, which as you learned in Chapter 1, raises blood pressure. If this form of high blood pressure doesn't respond to drug treatment or if kidney function is severely impaired, the obstruction may be opened with catheters and stents like those used in treating narrowed coronary arteries.

Sometimes, narrowed renal arteries can be diagnosed with a stethoscope; the turbulent blood flow produces distinctive sounds. Narrowed arteries and changes in your kidneys can also be detected through imaging involving ultrasound, angiography, CT and MRI.

Thyroid disorders: An uncommon cause

The thyroid gland regulates your metabolism, from how fast your heart beats to how quickly you burn calories. As long as your thyroid gland produces the right amount of the hormone thyroxine, your metabolism functions as it should.

But sometimes the gland produces too much or too little thyroxine, upsetting the balance of chemical reactions in your body. You may have hyperthyroidism, which is overproduction of thyroxine. This may raise your systolic blood pressure and heart rate.

Or you may have hypothyroidism, which is when the body produces too little thyroxine. This can also raise blood pressure.

Rare causes of secondary hypertension

On rare occasions, other issues with the adrenal gland or a problem with the aorta can lead to high blood pressure. Here's more on these conditions.

Pheochromocytoma

This condition occurs when a tumor forms in the inner layer of an adrenal gland. The tumor, which can also occur in other parts of your body and in multiple locations, secretes the hormones epinephrine and norepinephrine and other chemicals. Pheochromocytoma almost always causes noticeable signs and symptoms. If you have one of these tumors, you may have sudden and severe headaches, a pounding heartbeat and profuse sweating and paleness. These spells may last from minutes to an hour. They may happen daily or infrequently. Blood pressure is almost always much higher during a spell. It may also be high between spells.

You may have blood and urine tests and imaging with CT, MRI or isotopes to diagnose this condition. Genetic tests also may be helpful because this condition can run in families. The tumor is rarely cancerous and can be removed with surgery.

Cushing syndrome

Cortisol is produced in the adrenal glands. You learned how the adrenal glands work in Chapter 1. Sometimes, a growth on one of the adrenal glands produces excess cortisol. Alternately, a tumor on the pituitary gland at the base of the brain may send a signal to the adrenal glands to produce too much cortisol. Too much cortisol in the body can cause high blood pressure, among many other issues. Treatment for Cushing syndrome is directed toward reducing the excess amounts of cortisol.

Coarctation of the aorta

This condition involves a narrowing of the primary artery (aorta) from the heart.

THYROID GLAND

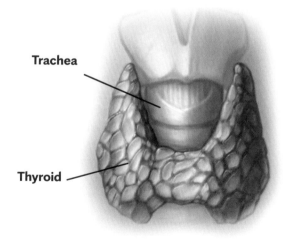

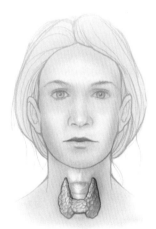

Abnormal hormone production in the butterfly-shaped thyroid gland can cause hyperthyroidism or hypothyroidism.

Trachea

Thyroid

It usually occurs in the part of the aorta in the chest and, rarely, in your belly. It's usually seen at birth, but occasionally a person may reach adulthood before it's detected.

A narrowed aorta results in high blood pressure in the arms and low blood pressure in the legs. A member of your health care team can detect this when feeling the artery in your groin and at your wrist at the same time. The pulse in your groin will be slightly delayed and less forceful than the pulse at your wrist. A chest X-ray and imaging with ultrasound or MRI can establish the diagnosis.

Coarctation is repaired with surgery. The narrowed portion of the aorta is removed and the ends of the vessel are rejoined. In some cases, angioplasty is used to stretch open the narrow section using a balloon on the end of a catheter (balloon dilatation). If angioplasty fails to permanently expand the area, a metallic stent may be inserted through a catheter to hold the area open.

Identifying secondary high blood pressure

Similar to essential high blood pressure, you may not know you have secondary high blood pressure until you've had an exam that confirms it. Generally, with the secondary form, symptoms associated with the underlying condition may be what brought you to your doctor's office.

If it's discovered that you have high blood pressure, your health care team will want to know details of your medical history as well as your family history. You'll also likely have tests to find evidence of heart attack, heart disease, hardening of the arteries, weight change, leg pain during exercise, weakness and fatigue. Your health care team will also check for signs and symptoms of conditions that can cause secondary high blood pressure.

WAYS YOU CAN TAKE CHARGE NOW

Though you can't change some high blood pressure risk factors, there's plenty that you can do to lower your blood pressure and prevent hypertension. You learned about the risk factors within your control earlier in this chapter. Here's a closer look at the steps you can take to improve in each area.

Adopt a healthy diet

A healthy diet emphasizes lower fat and sodium intake, more vegetables, fruits and fiber, and reduced calories. A healthy diet can reduce your blood pressure as much as some medications. It should be plant based — rich in vegetables and fruit — and include whole grains, beans, nuts, fish, lean sources of protein, and low-fat or fat-free dairy products. Unhealthy fats (saturated fat and trans fat), sodium and alcohol intake are limited. For more on a healthy diet, see Chapter 5 in this book.

Move more

Regular physical activity is important for your health in many ways, including for lowering blood pressure. It can reduce your risk of hypertension, help you manage high blood pressure and help blood pressure medication work more effectively. Work toward 150 minutes a week of moderate physical activity, 75 minutes a week of vigorous physical activity or a combination of the two. To lose weight or maintain weight loss, work toward getting 300 minutes a week of moderate physical activity.

In addition to regular physical activity, try to limit the time you spend sitting. The more you sit, the greater your health risks. Learn more in Chapter 6.

Reach, maintain a healthy weight

Changes in weight and blood pressure often go hand in hand. When weight increases, blood pressure often does, too. Likewise, as you lose weight, blood pressure usually goes down. Losing as little as 10 to 20 pounds can help lower your blood pressure and heart disease risk. Weight loss can also improve cholesterol levels and reduce the risk of heart attack, stroke, diabetes and arthritis.

What's the link between body weight and blood pressure? As you put on weight, you gain mostly fatty tissue. This tissue relies on the nutrients in your blood to survive. As the demand for nutrients increases, the amount of circulating blood increases. More blood traveling through your arteries means greater pressure on the artery walls. Fatty tissue also is an active endocrine organ that produces substances having local and generalized effects on

blood vessels, kidneys and the heart. Another reason why blood pressure often increases when you're overweight is that additional weight typically raises your insulin level. More insulin is associated with the retention of sodium and water, which raises blood volume. In addition, excess body weight can increase your heart rate and reduce the capacity of your blood vessels to transport blood. Both factors can raise blood pressure.

Find your healthy weight

A healthy weight means you have the right amount of body fat in relation to your overall body mass. Guidelines from the American College of Cardiology, The Obesity Society and the American Heart Association take a threefold approach to determining a healthy weight. This approach is based on the following components:
• Body mass index
• Waist circumference
• Risk factors for diseases and conditions associated with obesity

The following do-it-yourself evaluations can tell you whether you could benefit from losing a few pounds. Doing so can help you control your blood pressure and lessen the risk of other health problems.

Body mass index

Body mass index (BMI) is a standard formula that factors in your weight and height in determining whether you have a healthy or unhealthy percentage of body fat. Except in very muscular people such as athletes, this measurement correlates well with total body fat.

To determine your BMI, locate your height on the chart on page 43 and follow it across until you reach the weight nearest yours. Look for the number at the top of the column to find your BMI. If your weight is less than the weight nearest yours, your BMI may be slightly less. If your weight is greater than the weight nearest yours, your BMI may be slightly greater.

A BMI of 18.5 to 24.9 is considered healthy. A BMI of 25 to 29.9 signifies overweight, and a BMI of 30 or more indicates obesity. If your BMI is 25 or greater, your risk of developing a weight-related disease such as hypertension is higher.

For Asians, a BMI of 23 or greater may indicate an increased risk of health problems; a BMI of at least 27.5 indicates even higher risk.

Waist circumference

This measurement, used in combination with your BMI, is also important in evaluating a healthy weight. It indicates where most of your fat is located.

In short, the bigger your waistline, the greater your health risks. Carrying weight around the belly increases your risk of high blood pressure, diabetes, abnormal cholesterol levels, metabolic syndrome, coronary artery disease, stroke and some types of cancer. If you carry weight around your hips, your risk of these conditions isn't as high.

To determine whether you have too much weight around your belly, measure your waist circumference. Place a tape measure around your bare abdomen, just above your hipbone. Make sure that the tape is parallel to the floor and that it's snug but doesn't compress your skin. Relax, exhale and measure your waist.

Women with a waist circumference of more than 35 inches and men with a waist circumference of more than 40 inches have increased health risks.

Other considerations

Numbers alone aren't enough. It's also important to know how likely it is that you will have a disease or condition that's linked to being overweight. Consider the following questions:

- Do you have a condition such as high blood pressure, arthritis or type 2 diabetes that would improve if you lost weight?
- Do you have a family history of a weight-related illness, such as high blood pressure, type 2 diabetes, high cholesterol, high triglycerides or sleep apnea?
- Do you have any other risk factors, such as smoking or inactivity?

Think of BMI and waist measurement as snapshots of your current health status. Your medical history helps provide a more complete picture by revealing more

WHAT'S YOUR BMI?

You can determine your body mass index (BMI) by finding your height and weight on this chart. A BMI of 18.5 to 24.9 is considered normal. This means your weight is at a level at which it doesn't pose risks to your health. People with a BMI under 18.5 are considered underweight. People with a BMI between 25 and 29.9 are considered overweight. People with a BMI of 30 or greater are considered obese.

Healthy			Overweight					Obese				
BMI	19	24	25	26	27	28	29	30	35	40	45	50
Height	Weight in pounds											
4'10"	91	115	119	124	129	134	138	143	167	191	215	239
4'11"	94	119	124	128	133	138	143	148	173	198	222	247
5'0"	97	123	128	133	138	143	148	153	179	204	230	255
5'1"	100	127	132	137	143	148	153	158	185	211	238	264
5'2"	104	131	136	142	147	153	158	164	191	218	246	273
5'3"	107	135	141	146	152	158	163	169	197	225	254	282
5'4"	110	140	145	151	157	163	169	174	204	232	262	291
5'5"	114	144	150	156	162	168	174	180	210	240	270	300
5'6"	118	148	155	161	167	173	179	186	216	247	278	309
5'7"	121	153	159	166	172	178	185	191	223	255	287	319
5'8"	125	158	164	171	177	184	190	197	230	262	295	328
5'9"	128	162	169	176	182	189	196	203	236	270	304	338
5'10"	132	167	174	181	188	195	202	209	243	278	313	348
5'11"	136	172	179	186	193	200	208	215	250	286	322	358
6'0"	140	177	184	191	199	206	213	221	258	294	331	368
6'1"	144	182	189	197	204	212	219	227	265	302	340	378
6'2"	148	186	194	202	210	218	225	233	272	311	350	389
6'3"	152	192	200	208	216	224	232	240	279	319	359	399
6'4"	156	197	205	213	221	230	238	246	287	328	369	410

National Institutes of Health, 1998.

Note: Asians with a BMI of 33 or higher may have an increased risk of health problems.

about your risk of being overweight or developing weight-related diseases.

Add up the results

If your BMI shows you're not overweight and you're not carrying too much weight around your belly, there's likely no health advantage to changing your weight. You can consider your weight to be healthy.

If your BMI is between 25 and 29.9, you may benefit from losing a few pounds, particularly if your waist circumference exceeds healthy guidelines or you answered yes to at least one of the medical history questions. Talk to your health care team about your options.

If your BMI is 30 or more, losing some weight will likely improve your health and reduce your risk of developing a weight-related illness.

Keys to successful weight loss

Plenty of people successfully lose weight and keep it off, and you can be one of them. Use these guidelines to lose weight safely and keep the pounds off for good.

Don't starve yourself

Extremely low-calorie diets and special food combinations aren't the answer to long-term weight control. Eating less than 1,200 calories makes it hard for your body to get enough nutrients. It also promotes temporary loss of fluids and of healthy muscle rather than fat loss.

KEY POINTS

- There are two forms of high blood pressure, primary and secondary. The cause of essential high blood pressure isn't known. Secondary high blood pressure results from an underlying illness or condition.
- Certain genetic and lifestyle factors place you at increased risk of developing high blood pressure. Generally, the more of these factors you have, the greater your risk.
- You may be able to prevent high blood pressure by eliminating or reducing certain risk factors that you can change. These include losing weight if you need to, maintaining a healthy weight, getting regular physical activity, keeping stress levels manageable, and adopting a healthy diet that's low in sodium and alcohol intake and high in potassium.
- If you have elevated blood pressure, reducing it can help keep you from developing high blood pressure, cardiovascular disease and other diseases.

Change gradually

The first rule of change is to not change too quickly — it's not a race. You're trying to develop a whole new lifestyle. This doesn't happen overnight.

Set realistic goals

Aim to try to lose no more than 1 to 2 pounds a week.

Get and stay active

Physical activity is the most important factor related to long-term weight loss. Exercise helps you lose body fat and build muscle, making it easier to maintain weight loss.

Maintain your progress

Don't let minor setbacks weaken your resolve to lose weight. When a lapse in your diet or exercise happens, rethink what you can do to reinsert the healthy behavior back in your daily routine.

WHY ACT NOW?

You may wonder why it's so important to take steps to prevent high blood pressure. Why not simply wait for the condition to develop and then treat it, possibly with a little better diet and a little more activity?

There are many reasons why it's better to act now instead of waiting for later.

Generally, the younger you are when you try to change your lifestyle, the better your chances are of succeeding at it. The longer you're able to maintain a healthy weight, the lower your risk of weight-related diseases.

Even successful blood pressure treatment may not completely reverse the changes to your heart and arteries. It's better to prevent the damage from ever happening.

How high blood pressure is diagnosed

Unlike many other chronic health conditions, high blood pressure rarely produces signs and symptoms to warn you that something is wrong. Most people who have high blood pressure, even when they've had it for a long time and it's uncontrolled, look and feel just fine.

During routine medical examinations is when most people learn that their blood pressure is too high. That's why it's important to have your blood pressure checked at least once every two years. Otherwise, vital organs, such as your heart and kidneys, could be damaged by high blood pressure without you even knowing it.

Fortunately, diagnosing high blood pressure is a relatively straightforward process. It generally involves several measurements taken in a medical office over a period of several weeks or months.

This process confirms whether an initial high reading was simply a temporary change or if it represents what has become your regular level.

As part of the process, you'll likely answer questions about your health and your family's health, have a physical exam, and get routine lab tests. These steps are taken to determine whether any organs have been damaged because of high pressure levels. Treating high blood pressure early may also prevent additional health problems from developing. Results from the physical exam and lab tests also help guide treatment. (See "Key questions to answer" starting on page 49.)

Two methods for reducing and controlling high blood pressure are lifestyle changes and medication. Whether you'll need medication depends on your blood pressure level, the presence of other health conditions that increase your risk of heart disease, and whether any organ damage has occurred.

TAKING A BLOOD PRESSURE READING

Measuring blood pressure is a simple procedure that you can learn to do. Readings are typically taken with an electronic sphygmomanometer, which includes a fully automatic monitor.

These electronic units inflate and deflate the cuff, detect systolic and diastolic pressures by sensing vibrations in the wall of the artery, and then display blood pressure measurements on a digital screen. To get accurate readings, the inflatable part of the blood pressure cuff should cover about half the distance around your upper arm, approximately 80% of the area from your elbow to your shoulder.

Monitoring blood pressure at home is advised. Chapter 10 provides instructions on how to take your blood pressure

ELECTRONIC MONITORS

You can use an electronic monitor at home to check your blood pressure. Learn more about electronic blood pressure monitors and how to use them in Chapter 10.

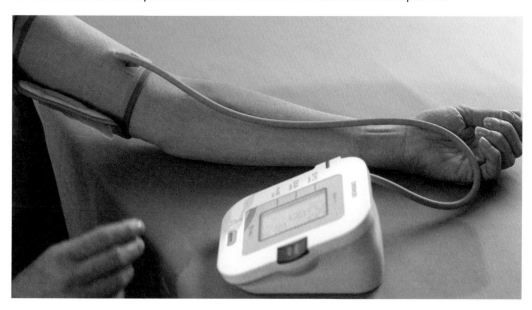

yourself, as well as advice on electronic blood pressure monitors.

Making certain

A blood pressure reading of 120/80 millimeters of mercury (mm Hg) or higher in a medical office is considered elevated, and a reading of 130/80 mm Hg or above is considered high. But a single reading usually isn't enough to diagnose hypertension. Blood pressure varies throughout the day, so it's best to get many readings under similar circumstances.

Only if the reading is extremely high — a systolic pressure of 180 mm Hg or higher or a diastolic pressure of 120 mm Hg or higher — is a diagnosis made based on a single measurement.

FALSE READINGS

Sometimes, blood pressure measurements can produce false high readings. This happens most often among older adults with damaged arteries that have become very stiff, and it's different from what's known as white coat hypertension (see page 50). Although many people with stiff arteries have high blood pressure, it may not be as high as the measurements show.

The false readings occur because it's hard for rigid arteries to collapse. When a blood pressure measurement is taken, the cuff may not be able to collapse the brachial artery until the cuff has been inflated to extremely high pressure. And when pressure in the cuff is released, stiffness causes the artery to open faster than it should, which gives an incorrect reading.

Your health care team often can tell whether you have this condition, called pseudohypertension, by feeling your forearm. Usually, when a blood pressure cuff collapses your brachial artery, the person taking your blood pressure can't feel the arteries in your forearm below the cuff.

Stiff arteries in the forearm, however, remain open and can be felt even when no blood is flowing through them. People with this condition may find that electronic devices also fail to give accurate readings. In this case, your blood pressure will be treated more cautiously and your health care team will look for symptoms that might occur if your blood pressure is overtreated. Fortunately, this is an uncommon situation.

Generally, a diagnosis of high blood pressure is made after at least two visits with your health care team in which your blood pressure is measured at least twice during each visit. In all, you'll have at least four measurements taken. You may also be diagnosed with high blood pressure if measurements taken at home are elevated on several occasions.

If the average of the measurements — in a medical office or at home — shows your blood pressure to be 130/80 mm Hg or higher, you have high blood pressure.

As you prepare to have your blood pressure tested, keep these tips in mind to ensure an accurate reading:
- Don't smoke, eat a big meal or drink caffeine or alcohol for at least 30 minutes before taking your blood pressure. You'll also want to make sure your bladder is empty. All of these factors can change blood pressure for a period of time.
- Give yourself plenty of time to make it to your appointment. Rushing around can cause stress, and this can temporarily increase your blood pressure.
- Before you have your blood pressure measured, sit comfortably and quietly for 5 minutes with your back supported and both feet flat on the floor.
- When having your blood pressure taken, don't talk. Talking can elevate blood pressure. Some offices now have an automatic device that takes readings every few minutes while you're alone, quiet and seated properly.

KEY QUESTIONS TO ANSWER

Your medical history, a complete physical exam and lab tests can help provide answers to these questions:
- Has your high blood pressure damaged any organs?
- Is your high blood pressure primary (essential) or secondary? Although secondary high blood pressure is uncommon, it's important to consider secondary causes. As you learned earlier, some of these conditions are

WHY DO I NEED TO RETURN FOR MORE BLOOD PRESSURE READINGS AFTER MY FIRST VISIT?

Let's say that at a routine medical exam, your blood pressure reading was above 130/80 mm Hg. Unless your blood pressure was extremely high (180/120 mm Hg or higher), you'll need to return for additional checks. That's because many factors can affect your blood pressure, and measurements vary widely throughout the day and from day to day. At least two measurements are taken at each of your next visits, generally under the same circumstances. A fair gauge of your regular blood pressure is the average of these measurements from at least two visits.

WHITE COAT HYPERTENSION AND MASKED HYPERTENSION

Often, people have higher blood pressure readings in a medical office than they do when they're not. This condition, called white coat hypertension or isolated clinic hypertension, occurs in around 14% to almost 38% of people with high blood pressure measured in a clinic setting.

For other people, the opposite holds true. Their blood pressure is consistently higher when they're at home or at work than it is in a medical office. This condition is called masked hypertension. It may occur for many reasons. For example, the calm, quiet environment of a medical office may be less stressful than the other environments they live in.

If your health care team thinks your high blood pressure is white coat hypertension, you may need to keep track of your blood pressure away from a medical setting. For both white coat and masked hypertension, you may need to wear a portable device (ambulatory monitor) that measures your blood pressure periodically over a 24-hour period while you go about your regular activities. For either condition, this method can generally provide you with a more realistic and accurate assessment of your blood pressure.

Automated machines in stores and shopping malls that measure blood pressure aren't recommended alternatives. These machines aren't accurate enough, and they often have cuffs that don't fit well. Plus, the settings where these machines are located — which can have a huge impact on blood pressure readings — aren't controlled and, in fact, can be chaotic.

Conventional medical thought was that white coat hypertension was harmless, not requiring treatment. But 1 to 3 out of 100 people per year with white coat hypertension will develop sustained high blood pressure. Research suggests that masked hypertension poses the same risks as sustained high blood pressure.

If you have white coat hypertension, your health care team may recommend making lifestyle changes to prevent sustained hypertension and monitoring blood pressure at home to identify hypertension if it develops.

If you have masked hypertension, you'll be treated just as you would if you had sustained hypertension.

treatable, allowing you to reduce blood pressure, possibly without medication.
- Do you have other risk factors that increase your chances of having a heart attack or stroke, such as tobacco use, too much weight, an inactive lifestyle, high blood cholesterol or diabetes?

If it's unclear whether you have high blood pressure or elevated blood pressure, these evaluations can help confirm the diagnosis and guide treatment decisions for the condition.

Medical history

Your medical history may point to a particular factor or event that has triggered the increase in blood pressure. This history can also help your health care team assess your risk of other health conditions. You may be asked about the following:
- Previous blood pressure readings
- Personal history of heart disease, kidney disease, high cholesterol, diabetes and sleep apnea (such as snoring, restless sleep or daytime sleepiness)
- Family history of high blood pressure, heart attack, stroke, kidney disease, diabetes, high cholesterol or early (premature) death
- Signs and symptoms that may suggest secondary high blood pressure, such as spells of looking very pale, rapid heart rate, intolerance of heat or unexplained weight loss

You may also be asked questions about the following:

- Alcohol use
- Diet and use of salt (sodium)
- Medications you're currently taking
- Tobacco use
- Changes in weight
- Caffeine use
- Activity level

Tell your health care team about all medications you take — both prescription and over the counter, as well as illicit drugs and herbal and nutritional supplements. Be sure to mention any drugs that you've reacted badly to.

Some drugs can increase blood pressure, while others don't react well with some blood pressure medications and can lead to dangerous interactions. As for supplements, more research is needed regarding the health effects of many of them. That's why it's important to compile a list of all of the medications and supplements you take, including drug names and dosages. If you don't have a list, bring the original containers with you to your next visit with your health care team. Learn more about medications in Chapter 8.

Keep in mind that blood pressure naturally rises and falls over a 24-hour period. Diet, activities, emotions and other factors also affect blood pressure. These variations must be taken into account as you and your health care team consider your use of medications.

Physical exam

A member of your health care team will examine your body for signs of organ damage and check for signs of a possible secondary cause for the blood pressure increase.

For signs of organ damage, your health care team may look for:

Eye changes

Damage to the blood vessels in the eyes is a strong indicator that blood vessels elsewhere in the body have been damaged by high pressure (see images on page 24). This may also indicate an increased risk of heart disease. Your health care team may look for signs such as narrowed or leaky blood vessels in the eyes.

Heart issues

A fast heart rate, a heart that's enlarged in size, an unusual heartbeat rhythm or a click or murmur in the sounds of the heart can signal possible heart disease.

Turbulent blood flow

When a blood vessel narrows, it can cause turbulent blood flow called a bruit (bru-we). It most often occurs in the carotid arteries in the neck and the major arteries in the belly.

Decreased blood pressure when you stand

A side effect of some blood pressure medications is fainting or dizziness upon standing (postural hypotension). Such dizziness is also a complication of diabetes. It's common in older adults, particularly after meals, whether or not they have diabetes.

Aortic aneurysm

An aneurysm can form at a weak spot in the wall of the aorta. A member of your health care team may feel it while examining your belly. A stethoscope also may pick up the sound of blood pulsing through the weakened blood vessel. In addition to high blood pressure, smoking is a major risk factor for these aneurysms.

Weakened pulse

A weak pulse in the groin, lower legs and ankles can signal artery damage.

Reduced blood pressure in your ankles

This can result from narrowed or diseased blood vessels in the legs.

Swelling

A buildup of fluid in the lower legs and ankles is a common sign of heart or kidney failure.

Enlarged kidneys or thyroid gland

If either of these organs becomes enlarged, it may indicate secondary high blood pressure from another condition.

High blood pressure can, at times, be hard to diagnose. If your health care team isn't sure whether you have high blood pressure and if so, how severe it is, you'll likely need to wear a special device known as an ambulatory monitor. This kind of monitoring is recommended to confirm whether you have hypertension.

This device is a portable blood pressure monitor that you can wear for a day. It includes an inflatable cuff that fits around your arm and a small monitoring unit that hangs at your waist using a strap over your shoulder. A thin tube connecting the monitor to the cuff may be secured to your skin with tape to prevent it from twisting or disconnecting.

The monitor is programmed to take your blood pressure about every 15 to 20 minutes during the day and every 30 to 60 minutes during sleep over a period of 24 hours. The device is fully automatic. At selected times, it pumps up the blood pressure cuff, deflates it, takes a reading and stores the information in its memory.

You may be a candidate for ambulatory monitoring if you have white coat hypertension (your blood pressure readings are higher than they should be, but only at medical checkups) or masked hypertension (you show complications of high blood pressure but have normal blood pressure readings at medical checkups). Ambulatory monitoring can also be helpful if your blood pressure rises and lowers over a wide range or if your blood pressure isn't responding to medications. Monitoring your blood pressure over 24 hours can help predict your risk of heart disease caused by high blood pressure. If you're under age 50, your 24-hour diastolic blood pressure is the most important in determining your heart disease risk. For adults older than age 50, systolic blood pressure is the most important. Ambulatory monitoring over 24 hours also can help detect secondary hypertension caused, for example, by sleep apnea.

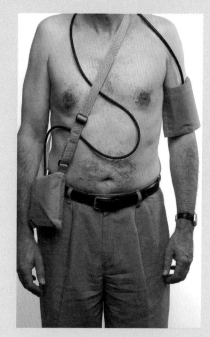

While wearing the monitor, you'll want to keep a journal that lists your daily activities and the times you did them, as well as the times you took medications, and any periods of stress, strong emotions or pain. By comparing the journal entries with your blood pressure readings from the ambulatory monitor, your health care team may note where certain events or lifestyle factors are linked to changes in your blood pressure.

Routine tests

The following tests are often included in a routine evaluation for high blood pressure:

Weight

Being overweight or obese may play a role in raising blood pressure. Weight usually is taken as part of a general office visit. You may have your body mass index (BMI) calculated to determine whether you're at a normal weight for your height (see pages 41-44). You may also have your waist measured to see if you're carrying too much weight around your belly (see page 42).

Complete blood cell count

This test reveals white and red blood cell counts that are higher or lower than they should be. Its purpose is to ensure that you don't have certain health conditions you may not be aware of, such as a low red blood cell count, called anemia.

Blood chemistry

The levels of sodium and potassium in your blood are measured. Blood may also be tested for levels of the compound creatinine, which can indicate damage to the kidneys.

Other common blood tests include measurements of cholesterol-containing blood fats (lipid profile). The higher the total blood cholesterol level and the lower the high-density lipoprotein (HDL, or "good") cholesterol level, the greater the risk of cardiovascular disease and metabolic syndrome.

A higher level of low-density lipoprotein (LDL, or "bad") cholesterol is a risk factor for cardiovascular disease. It builds up in the walls of the arteries, making them hard and narrowed.

The level of glucose (sugar) in the blood also may be measured to check for diabetes.

Urinalysis

The presence of protein or red blood cells in urine can indicate kidney damage. A form of protein in the urine, called microalbuminuria, also can signal early stage kidney disease — a risk factor for future heart disease. In addition, urine may be tested for the presence of sugar (glucose) resulting from diabetes. Diabetes increases the risk of damage that hypertension causes to the cardiovascular system.

Electrocardiography

The heart's electrical activity is monitored to check for rhythm issues or signs of damage, such as an enlarged heart or lack of blood supply. Changes in the heart's electrical activity are recorded on an electrocardiogram (ECG), which can also show high or low levels of potassium.

Additional tests

If your physical exam and lab tests don't show any issues, you probably won't have to have additional tests. However, further tests may be necessary if you have:
- Very high blood pressure (180 mm Hg or higher/120 mm Hg or higher).
- Sudden onset of high blood pressure or a sharp increase in your usual blood pressure level.
- Low blood potassium level.
- Sound of turbulent blood flow (bruit) heard over an artery.
- Evidence of kidney problems.
- Evidence of heart problems.
- Indications of an abdominal aortic aneurysm.
- Evidence of hormonal disorders.

If narrowed arteries are interrupting blood flow, imaging tests can identify the location and severity of the problem:

Angiography

During this procedure, a dye that's highly visible to an X-ray machine is injected into blood vessels. The X-ray machine rapidly takes a series of images (angiograms) that reveal hidden or subtle features of your arteries.

Magnetic resonance angiography (MRA)

Rather than using X-rays to produce an image, magnetic resonance imaging uses magnetic fields and radio waves. The device detects and stores small energy signals emitted by the atoms that make up body tissue. A computer program creates images based on this information.

Ultrasonography

This procedure uses high-frequency sound waves to track the function of the

COMPUTERIZED TOMOGRAPHY

A computerized tomography (CT) scan involves taking multiple, highly specialized X-rays of an organ such as the heart. With the help of computer programs, highly detailed images of the heart and blood vessels can be created.

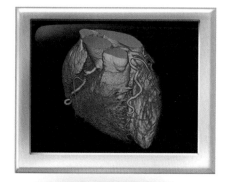

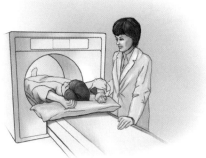

circulatory system. The waves bounce off internal structures and back to a transducer, which converts the reflected waves into a distinct image.

If your health care team suspects that you may have a shrunken kidney, an abdominal aortic aneurysm or an adrenal gland tumor, additional tests may include:

Magnetic resonance imaging (MRI)

This procedure is based on the same principles as the MRA, but MRI provides detailed images of organs rather than blood vessels.

Computerized tomography (CT) scan

The image produced in a CT scan is generated by an X-ray beam, but this technology provides much more information than an ordinary X-ray. That's because the doughnut-shaped machine contains a rotating scanner that emits a series of beams from all angles around your body.

A computer gathers these X-ray signals and processes them into highly detailed, 3D images of the internal organs (see images on the bottom of page 55).

Nuclear scanning

After radioactive material is injected into a vein, nuclear images are taken that show the material passing through a specific location or organ. Nuclear scans are used to monitor blood flow and to determine the size and function of organs.

CHAPTER

What the numbers mean

4

High blood pressure treatment is tailored to each person's needs. The treatment that works for someone else may not be the best fit for you. Your medical history, physical exam and lab tests are used to determine an effective, personalized plan.

There are two basic approaches to lowering high blood pressure: adopting healthy lifestyle habits and taking medications. Depending on your health and risk factors, lifestyle changes may include losing weight, getting more active, making diet changes, quitting smoking, limiting alcohol and managing stress.

In terms of medications, there are several types to choose from. Each type affects blood pressure in different ways. It's important not to share the drugs prescribed for you with anyone else. Someone else's medication may not be the

same type as yours or the dosage may be different.

LATEST GUIDELINES

In November 2017, the American College of Cardiology and the American Heart Association, working with nine other U.S. health care organizations, released a new guideline for the prevention, detection, evaluation and management of high blood pressure. The new guideline — the first comprehensive U.S. national blood pressure guideline since 2003 — lowered the threshold of what is defined as high blood pressure. The change was made to account for new data indicating that complications can occur at lower blood pressure levels and that controlling blood pressure to lower levels provides added protection from cardiovascular damage.

Treatment for elevated blood pressure and hypertension depends on several factors, including your systolic and diastolic blood pressure levels and whether you have additional heart disease risk factors, which put you at a higher risk of heart attack and stroke.

While the treatment goal is the same — to lower your blood pressure — your number of risk factors determines when blood pressure drugs will be used to lower blood pressure alongside lifestyle changes. That's because the more factors you have, the greater the risk of complications, such as heart attack and stroke. Special attention will be given to addressing risk factors you can change, such as tobacco use, high cholesterol levels and diabetes.

The 2017 guideline recommends reducing blood pressure to less than 130/80 millimeters of mercury (mm Hg) if you have a history of heart disease, stroke, kidney disease or diabetes. If you don't have any of these conditions, aim for a blood pressure goal of less than 130/80 mm Hg. A slightly higher reading may be OK while you work on lifestyle changes.

If lifestyle changes alone can't lower your blood pressure to recommended levels, medication should be considered. If your

blood pressure is within the range for stage 2 hypertension — a systolic reading of 140 mm Hg or higher or a diastolic reading of 90 mm Hg or higher — or you have other cardiovascular risk factors, you may need to start taking medication right away.

The most important message here is to work with your health care team to develop a treatment plan that's suited to your specific situation. There are many opinions about which blood pressure goals are best to reach for optimal health, especially for older adults and those who have kidney disease or diabetes. And not all experts agree on the blood pressure level that's best for every person. When setting your blood pressure goal, you and your health care team should consider:
- Your overall health.
- Your risk of heart disease, stroke and kidney disease.
- Any other medical conditions you have.
- Prescription and over-the-counter therapies you're taking.
- Your gender and ethnicity.

Together, you and your health care team can decide on your treatment goal and medications you should take. Your plan should fit your lifestyle, give you good quality of life, and help you reduce your risk of heart disease, stroke and other consequences of high blood pressure.

Elevated blood pressure

If your systolic pressure (top number) is between 120 and 129 mm Hg and your diastolic pressure (bottom number) is less

GUIDELINES FOR TREATMENT

Blood pressure goals for individuals with high blood pressure

Adults with cardiovascular disease or other risk factors	Less than 130/80 mm Hg is recommended
Healthy adults at low risk of complications	Aim for less than 130/80 mm Hg

Habits that can help high blood pressure treatment	Risks to your body from untreated or poorly treated high blood pressure
• Eat a healthy diet, which includes limiting sodium and getting enough potassium • Get regular physical activity • Reach and maintain a healthy weight • Manage stress • Avoid tobacco smoke • If you drink, limit alcohol	• Damage to the heart and coronary arteries • Stroke • Kidney damage • Vision loss • Erectile dysfunction (impotence, or ED) • Memory loss • Fluid in the lungs • Chest pain (angina) • Peripheral artery disease

Source: Whelton PK, et al. 2017. Guideline for the Prevention, Detection, Evaluation, and Management of High Blood Pressure in Adults.

DISEASE PROGRESS: THE NUMBERS ARE MIXED

Since 1972, when the National Heart, Lung, and Blood Institute began an intensive education campaign, there has been steady improvement in awareness, treatment and control of high blood pressure. As a result, death and disability attributed to the disease have declined significantly. This is considered one of the best public health achievements in the 20th century.

During the early 1990s, however, those dramatic improvements slowed. The reasons for the slowdown are unclear. However, an increase in obesity and lack of exercise may be important factors.

The number of adults considered to be overweight or obese continues to increase. A report by the U.S. Surgeon General also found that only about 1 in 5 adults over age 18 met the U.S. physical activity guidelines for aerobic activity and strength training.

Another important factor may be complacency. Above-normal blood pressure too often may be overlooked — both by health care providers and their patients — as being "almost" in control and therefore not of great concern.

Although general blood pressure goals have changed, that doesn't mean they're any less important to reach. If your blood pressure is higher than your recommended goal, talk to your health care team about it. If you've lowered your blood pressure but still haven't reached your goal, get advice from your health care team about why this is and how you can create a plan to reach your blood pressure goal.

There is also good news. Data gathered in a review article, as well as patient care data from managed care organizations and the Department of Veterans Affairs, show positive improvement among people with high blood pressure. The control rate in a Veterans Affairs study population improved from 43% to almost 77% in a 10-year period. These improvements were seen in all age and ethnic groups and in both men and women.

than 80 mm Hg, you have elevated blood pressure.

Having elevated blood pressure means that you have a higher risk of developing hypertension and cardiovascular complications. Lifestyle changes such as a healthier diet and more exercise may reduce your blood pressure.

Stage 1 hypertension

If your systolic pressure (top number) is between 130 and 139 mm Hg or your diastolic pressure (bottom number) is between 80 and 89 mm Hg, you have stage 1 hypertension.

Lifestyle changes are part of the first-line treatment for stage 1 hypertension. You'll likely also need medication to bring your blood pressure under control. Angiotensin-converting enzyme (ACE) inhibitors, angiotensin II receptor blockers (ARBs), calcium channel blockers (CCBs) and thiazide diuretics are all commonly recommended first-choice medications, including for those who have diabetes.

Stage 2 hypertension

If your systolic pressure is 140 mm Hg or higher or your diastolic pressure is 90 mm Hg or higher, you have stage 2 hypertension.

People who have stage 2 hypertension are at the greatest risk of heart attack, stroke or other problems related to high blood pressure.

A combination of two blood pressure medications along with changes in lifestyle is typically recommended for stage 2 hypertension. Medications used to treat stage 2 hypertension may include a thiazide diuretic or a CCB in combination with an ACE inhibitor or ARB. Learn more about medications used to treat high blood pressure in Chapter 8.

Your treatment plan will include specific goals that take into account other factors in addition to your blood pressure level and unhealthy behaviors. For example, your health care team will consider your overall health and the other diseases and conditions you have when discussing your goals and treatment.

MEDICATION STILL REQUIRES LIFESTYLE CHANGES

Many people who take high blood pressure medication think that's all they have to do — that taking medication means they don't have to make lifestyle changes. But this isn't true.

Sometimes, medication can reduce blood pressure by only a certain amount. And that amount may not be enough to reach your blood pressure target level. For example, if you take in too much salt, your medication may not lower your blood pressure enough. Following a low-sodium diet, on the other hand, can help blood pressure medication work more effectively. Successfully making lifestyle changes in addition to taking medication often can help you reach your target blood pressure level.

In addition, if you can reach your blood pressure goal with medication, making lifestyle changes may help reduce the amount of medication you need. Less medication usually means less cost.

Also, with many blood pressure-lowering drugs, side effects increase with higher doses, so a lower dose may mean fewer or less severe side effects.

Plus, lifestyle changes are important for everyone with high blood pressure. They reduce risk of stroke, heart attack, heart failure, kidney failure and dementia.

LEAN ON YOUR HEALTH CARE TEAM

Achieving your blood pressure goals requires your full involvement. Meet with

---

HOW DO I MANAGE LIFESTYLE CHANGES?

It can be overwhelming to try to adjust your diet, start exercising, lower stress, stop smoking and watch your alcohol intake all at once. Use these general pointers to help guide you and keep you on track:

First, keep your goals realistic. If you set your expectations too high or hold yourself to impossible goals, you're setting yourself up for failure. For example, don't expect to do a five-mile run as soon as you start jogging.

Second, don't try to change too quickly. This is not a race. You're trying to develop a new lifestyle, shedding habits you've probably followed for many years. This doesn't happen overnight.

Third, it's important that you enjoy the changes you're making. If you don't like what you're doing, it's unlikely you'll stick with it.

Fourth, you will lapse here and there. For example, travel or work deadlines may cause you to eat poorly and not exercise. When this happens, don't get discouraged — just get back on your plan. It's all part of the process.

Fifth and finally, stay focused on your health. Remember that being healthy allows you to be energetic, strong and active and to experience the quality of life you want to achieve. Think of all the reasons you're making these changes. They'll keep you going all along the way, especially when you face struggles and setbacks. They represent the inner drive that keeps you moving forward with the healthy changes you set out to make.

If you're diagnosed with high blood pressure or considered to be at high risk for the condition, you may need to make fundamental changes to your lifestyle. This makes you an active participant in your health care.

Recognize that it takes a team effort to treat high blood pressure. You can't do it alone, and you can't depend on your health care team to do it for you. Everyone working together and supporting you, including family and friends, can help you achieve your goals.

your health care team regularly to assess your progress and adjust your treatment plan. Reaching your goal sooner results in lower risk of cardiovascular events occurring, so don't wait for more than a few months for lifestyle changes or medications to work.

If your medication causes side effects, talk to your health care team about cutting back on the dosage to reduce them. Some people who've significantly changed their lifestyles have been able to stop taking medications entirely.

You can live a long and healthy life with high blood pressure. But to do so, it's important to recognize that high blood pressure is a serious condition — and it's also one that you can bring under control.

5

How diet and weight loss help

Of all the factors that influence blood pressure, your diet is one that you can do a lot about. You can't change your genes or stop aging, but you can decide what food to put on your plate and how much to eat. By choosing healthy foods in the right amounts, you can lower your blood pressure and keep it under better control.

A healthy diet, along with physical activity and other lifestyle changes, can lessen the chance that you'll need medication to treat high blood pressure. Or it may mean you'll take fewer medications or at a lower dose. And you may be able to avoid high blood pressure entirely. These changes can also help you reach and maintain a healthy weight, as weight is another important risk factor when it comes to high blood pressure.

The more you can do to eat well and keep your weight in check, the better off your blood pressure will be. This chapter will kick-start your efforts by helping you gauge your weight and eating habits and pinpoint areas in which you can improve. Every choice counts.

Start by taking the assessment on pages 66-67. In what areas are you doing well? Where can you improve?

Use what you learn from this simple quiz as inspiration for setting goals that will help you lower your blood pressure and enhance your overall health.

MAKE A 'DASH' TOWARD HEALTHY EATING

The basic premise of any healthy diet is this: It's plant based (rich in vegetables and fruits). It includes whole grains, beans, nuts and other legumes. It may include fish, lean meats, eggs and low-fat dairy products. It offers plenty of nutrients and fiber, while limiting unhealthy fats and cholesterol. It also limits calories, aiding in weight loss. Small shifts in any area can affect blood pressure.

Though there are many diets out there, the best one for lowering blood pressure is the DASH diet. Known officially as Dietary Approaches to Stop Hypertension (DASH), it provides a lifelong approach to healthy eating.

The DASH diet stems from several key studies that compared various eating plans. In the first study, people with or at risk of high blood pressure followed one of three diets: a "typical" American diet, the DASH diet or a diet that promoted fruits and vegetables but didn't limit dairy products or fat. Those who followed the DASH diet reduced their blood pressure significantly — and within two weeks. Black participants and those with high blood pressure experienced the most dramatic drops. The DASH diet also lowered levels of low-density lipoprotein (LDL, or "bad") cholesterol.

The initial DASH diet included about 3,000 milligrams (mg) daily of sodium — less than what most Americans consume on a daily basis. A follow-up study, called the DASH-Sodium study, found that consuming less salt lowered blood pressure even more. Those who consumed no more than 1,500 mg of sodium a day experienced the greatest reductions in blood pressure.

One study found that people with elevated blood pressure and stage 1 hypertension who combined the DASH diet with lifestyle changes that included weight loss, physical activity and reduced sodium and alcohol intake were able to achieve better blood pressure control.

In the OmniHeart Trial, researchers modified the DASH diet by replacing some carbohydrates with either more protein or more unsaturated fat. Both diets lowered blood pressure further and improved triglyceride and cholesterol levels, possibly reducing the risk of coronary artery disease.

Another eating plan that can help control high blood pressure is the Mediterranean diet. Rooted in the traditional diets of countries such as Greece and Italy, the Mediterranean diet includes generous amounts of fruits, vegetables, olive oil, legumes, nuts, pasta, rice and bread. Moderate amounts of fish, dairy products, wine and beans are part of this diet, and red meat is eaten only sparingly. Processed foods, often high in sodium, are eaten very little, if at all.

Compared with the DASH diet, the Mediterranean diet includes more unsaturated fats, mainly from the use of olive oil, nuts and fish. Considered heart-healthy, unsaturated fats don't raise blood cholesterol levels.

ARE YOUR WEIGHT AND EATING HABITS HEALTHY?

What's your BMI? (Use the chart on page 43.)

☐ Obese (1 point)
☐ Underweight or overweight (2 points)
☐ Healthy (3 points)

What's your waist measurement? A waist circumference of more than 35 inches for women and more than 40 inches for men indicates increased health risks.

☐ Considerably more than the recommended measurement (1 point)
☐ Slightly above the recommended measurement (2 points)
☐ At or below the recommended measurement (3 points)

Do you have a health condition that would improve if you lost weight?

☐ Yes (1 point)
☐ Possibly (2 points)
☐ No (3 points)

Do you eat for emotional reasons, such as when you feel anxious, depressed, stressed, angry or excited?

☐ Always or quite often (1 point)
☐ Sometimes (2 points)
☐ Never or not often (3 points)

How often do you sit down and eat three regularly scheduled meals?

☐ Never or not often (1 point)
☐ Sometimes (2 points)
☐ Always or most of the time (3 points)

How long does it generally take you to eat a meal?

☐ Five minutes or less (1 point)
☐ Between five and 20 minutes (2 points)
☐ 20 minutes or more (3 points)

Do you snack a lot or often have snacks in place of meals?

☐ Yes or quite often (1 point)
☐ Occasionally (2 points)
☐ No or not often (3 points)

»» How did you score?

To the right of the answer you chose is a point value: 1, 2 or 3 points. Add up the points from your answers for your total score.

A: If your total score was 18 to 21 points, congratulations! Your weight and eating habits appear to be healthy.

B: If your score was 13 to 17 points, you're on track, but you may benefit from losing a few pounds and improving some of your eating habits.

C: If your score was 7 to 12 points, work toward making a healthy weight and better eating habits your priorities.

To lower blood pressure and prevent hypertension, research shows that the best combination of dietary choices includes following a Mediterranean diet or the DASH diet, eating less saturated fat and total fat, getting plenty of potassium, and limiting sodium and alcohol.

How to follow the DASH diet

Following is a look at the DASH eating plan by food group. It offers a guide to which types and amounts of foods are best. The DASH diet focuses on foods rich in nutrients that can help lower blood pressure, including essential minerals such as potassium, calcium and magnesium. You'll learn why these minerals are important later in this chapter.

In addition to plentiful amounts of fruits and vegetables, DASH includes whole grains, low-fat dairy products, poultry, fish and nuts. This diet follows heart-healthy guidelines by limiting saturated fat and cholesterol, as well as reducing intake of red meat, sweets and sugary beverages.

The following sections provide more detail on the types of food to choose when following the DASH diet.

Whole grains: 6 to 8 servings

Whole grains include foods such as whole-wheat bread and pasta, oatmeal, brown rice, grits and unsalted popcorn. Whole grains provide more natural fiber and nutrients than do highly processed or refined grains, such as white rice and white bread. Choose plain, whole-grain yeast breads rather than quick breads, sweet rolls or other baked goods that have added fat.

»TIP: Whole-grain breads and pasta are naturally low in fat and calories. To keep bread low in fat and calories, be cautious about what type of spread you slather on it. Avoid cream and cheese sauces on pasta. Instead, opt for vegetable or tomato-based sauces.

Vegetables and fruits: 4 to 5 servings each

Eating more vegetables and fruits may be one of the best things you can do to improve your blood pressure and your overall health. In addition to being low in calories, vegetables and fruits provide fiber, potassium and other wholesome nutrients that help lower blood pressure. Fruits and vegetables also contain phytochemicals — substances that may help reduce the risk of heart disease and some cancers.

Eating more vegetables and fruits can also help you reduce calories without cutting back on the amount you eat. These foods have a low energy density, meaning there are few calories in a large volume of food. They fill your stomach without adding many pounds. The key is to eat vegetables and fruits plain or with a few herbs and spices and to avoid smothering them with high-fat dips or sauces.

Potatoes, corn and peas make up nearly half the vegetables in the typical American diet. It's time to think beyond the french fry. Top-rated vegetables include dark green vegetables, such as broccoli, Brussels sprouts and spinach. There are many nutritious selections to include, such as romaine lettuce, tomatoes, bell peppers, onions, carrots and avocados.

All fruits are nutritious. Choose a variety — cantaloupe, tangerines, oranges, grapefruit, varieties of berries, apricots, kiwi, apples, pears, peaches, pineapple and watermelon.

»TIP: With plenty of vegetables, fruits and whole grains, the DASH diet is high in fiber. But increasing your fiber intake can sometimes cause bloating and diarrhea. To avoid these problems, increase your consumption of these foods gradually. You can also try taking Beano, an over-the-counter dietary supplement that helps prevent gas.

Fat-free or low-fat milk and milk products: 2 to 3 servings

Dairy products provide calcium as well as vitamin D, which helps your body absorb calcium. Dairy products are also valuable sources of protein in your diet.

When choosing dairy products, choose low-fat or fat-free varieties and avoid whole-fat varieties. Select skim or low-fat (1%) milk and yogurt, and fat-free or low-fat or reduced-fat cheeses.

Because cheese is higher in sodium, be sure to stay within recommended amounts (1 serving is 1.5 ounces). In recipes, substitute lower fat dairy products, such as skim or low-fat milk, for higher fat items. Note, however, that reduced-fat cream cheese and sour cream are higher in sodium than are their higher fat counterparts, so use them prudently.

»TIP: If you're lactose intolerant and you have problems digesting dairy products, you may benefit from choosing foods containing the enzyme lactase. This can reduce or prevent the symptoms of lactose intolerance. You can also take lactase tablets before eating the foods. Or choose a plant-based dairy alternative that's either naturally rich in or fortified with calcium.

Lean meats, poultry and fish: 6 or fewer servings

These foods are rich sources of protein, B vitamins, magnesium, iron and zinc. Choose lean cuts of meat, such as tenderloin, round or sirloin, and trim away the fat. When preparing poultry, remove the skin to reduce fat by about half. Keep in mind that even lean varieties of meat contain plenty of fat and cholesterol, so it's important to try to limit all animal food sources.

Fish provides one of the healthiest animal protein sources. Some fish contain high amounts of omega-3 fatty acids, which may reduce the risk of coronary artery disease and sudden cardiac death and lower blood pressure.

»TIP: Choose fresh or frozen meat, poultry and fish rather than processed,

Food group	Daily servings*	Serving sizes
Whole grains	6 to 8	½ cup (3 oz./90 g) cooked rice, pasta or cereal
		1 oz. (30 g) ready-to-eat (dry) cereal (serving size varies depending on cereal type)
		1 slice bread
		½ English muffin
Vegetables	4 to 5	1 cup (2 oz./60 g) raw leafy vegetables
		½ cup (3 oz./90 g) cut-up raw or cooked vegetables
		1 small potato
		½ cup (4 fl. oz./120 g) vegetable juice
Fruits	4 to 5	1 medium fruit, such as apple or banana
		17 grapes
		½ cup (3 oz./60 g) fresh, frozen or canned fruit
		¼ cup (1½ oz./45 g) dried fruit, such as raisins
		½ cup (4 fl. oz./180 mL) 100% fruit juice
Fat-free or low-fat milk and milk products	2 to 3	1 cup (8 fl. oz./250 mL) milk or 1 cup (8 oz./250 g) low-fat yogurt or 1½ oz. (45 g) cheese

Food group	Daily servings*	Serving sizes
Lean meats, poultry and fish	6 or fewer	1 oz. (30 g) cooked meats, poultry or fish 1 egg (no more than 4 egg yolks a week); 2 egg whites equal 1 egg
Nuts, seeds and legumes	4 to 5 a week	⅓ cup (1½ oz./45 g) nuts 2 tablespoons (1 oz./32 g) peanut butter 2 tablespoons (½ oz./15 g) seeds ½ cup (3½ oz./100 g) cooked legumes (dry beans or peas)
Fats and oils	2 to 3	1 teaspoon soft margarine 1 teaspoon vegetable oil 1 tablespoon mayonnaise 2 tablespoons regular salad dressing
Sweets	5 or fewer a week	1 tablespoon sugar 1 tablespoon jelly or jam ½ cup sorbet or gelatin 1 cup lemonade

*The lower number of recommended servings provides about 1,600 calories, midrange provides about 2,000 calories and the higher number provides about 2,400 calories.

Most Americans need between 1,600 and 2,400 calories daily, depending on age, sex and activity level. To lower the number of calories on the DASH diet, see page 77, or talk to a registered dietitian.

The DASH eating plan may be found on the National Heart, Lung, and Blood Institute website at www.nhlbi.nih.gov.

smoked or cured products, which often contain more than 200 mg of sodium per serving. Broiling, roasting and poaching are the healthiest ways to prepare meat, poultry and fish. You can cook fish in parchment paper or foil to seal in flavor and juices.

Nuts, seeds and legumes: 4 to 5 servings a week

These foods range from almonds, peanuts, walnuts, hazelnuts, peanut butter and sunflower seeds to legumes such as beans, split peas and lentils. They're an excellent source of protein and they contain no cholesterol. They also provide a variety of nutrients, including magnesium and potassium, plus phytochemicals and fiber.

Nuts and seeds do contain fat, but most of that fat is unsaturated, the type that helps protect against coronary artery disease.

»TIP: Be careful about salted nuts. Choose products with less than 200 mg of sodium per serving.

CHOOSE FATS WISELY

Not all fats are created equal. Most plans for healthy eating, including the DASH diet, require sharp limits on saturated fat. Foods high in saturated fats include red meat, whole-fat dairy products, and tropical oils made from coconut, palm and palm kernels.

Another type of unhealthy fat is trans fat, which can raise your "bad" (LDL) cholesterol levels and increase your risk of cardiovascular disease. Trans fats are found in partially hydrogenated oil. Used in the past in many processed foods such as crackers, cookies and deep-fried foods, trans fats have mostly been replaced with tropical oils or another saturated fat. Check food labels to steer clear of these fats.

Healthier fats include monounsaturated fats — found in olive oil, canola oil, peanut oil, nuts and avocados — and omega-3 fatty acids. Fatty fish such as salmon, mackerel and herring contain high amounts of omega-3 fatty acids, while smaller amounts are found in soybeans, nuts, flaxseed and canola oil.

Omega-3 fatty acids help your heart by lowering your blood triglyceride level and reducing your risk of blood clots, artery-clogging plaques and sudden death from heart rhythm issues. They also lower blood pressure.

Fats and oils: 2 to 3 servings

Many people are surprised to learn that certain fats are essential for good health. Fats provide reserves of stored energy and play vital roles in different body processes.

Your consumption of fats should be limited to the monounsaturated varieties, and limited in general. All fats contain about 45 calories per teaspoon and are high in caloric density. That means there are a lot of calories in a small amount.

Animal products — meat, dairy products and eggs and foods made with them — are the main source of fat in the American diet. Vegetables, fruits and grains are relatively low in fat. Healthy fats include soft margarine and olive, canola, corn and safflower oils.

»TIP: Invest in nonstick pans to cook foods. If you normally add a tablespoon of vegetable oil to a skillet, you can save about 120 calories and 14 grams of fat by using a nonstick skillet instead. Vegetable oil cooking spray adds only about 1 gram of fat and just a few calories.

Sweets: 5 or fewer a week

Sweets are a high source of calories but offer little nutrition. They include candies, cookies, cakes, pies and other desserts. The table sugar you add to cereal, fruit and beverages counts, too.

You don't have to give up sweets entirely, but be smart about what you select and how much you eat. When you do eat sweets, choose items with natural sweetness rather than sugary treats made with oil or butter.

Best choices include fruit-based desserts and those made with whole grains. Try frozen grapes, grilled pineapple, baked apples or a fruit cobbler topped with rolled oats. If you enjoy chocolate, try 1 ounce of dark chocolate or unsweetened or lightly sweetened cocoa powder sprinkled on oatmeal or mixed with milk.

»TIP: Replace all or part of the sugar in recipes with cinnamon, nutmeg, vanilla and fruit to enhance sweetness.

REACH AND MAINTAIN A HEALTHY WEIGHT

Along with healthy eating habits, losing extra weight can lower your blood pressure significantly. Losing weight offers other benefits as well, such as a reduced risk of diabetes and heart disease.

Choosing healthy foods and getting regular physical activity, which you'll read about later, are the key elements for weight loss.

It's a simple formula: Burn more calories than you take in, and you'll lose weight. Though it sounds simple in theory, many people struggle to make it happen. If you find it hard to lose weight, know that you're not alone — and that with the right blend of healthy habits, you can lose weight and improve your health.

You don't have to lose a lot of weight to make a difference. Losing as little as 5 pounds may reduce your blood pressure to a healthier level. If you're overweight, losing 5% to 10% of your body weight may be a good goal. Once you've achieved that goal, you can try for another 5% to 10% if you need to lose more weight. Over time, these losses can add up to a significant improvement in your health.

The most successful way to lose weight is to change your eating and activity habits and slim down gradually. The DASH eating plan and regular physical activity can help you do this.

Find your starting point

As a first step, look at your current calorie balance. How many calories are you taking in, and how many calories are you burning through exercise? Once you establish this baseline, you can plan your adjustments, both in diet and exercise.

The number of calories your body uses to carry out basic functions is your basal metabolic rate, also known as metabolism. This is the number of calories your body uses for all its "hidden" functions, such as breathing, circulating blood, adjusting hormone levels and growing and repairing cells.

To determine your basal metabolic rate, visit www.MayoClinic.org and search "calorie calculator." You'll input your age, height, weight, gender and usual level of activity. The number of calories you get as a result is your basal metabolic rate —

the number of calories your body needs daily to function. If you take in more calories than this and don't burn enough of them, you'll gain weight. But if you reduce this calorie level by taking in fewer calories and burning more calories through physical activity, you'll lose weight.

Adjust your calorie balance

After you find your basal metabolic rate, you'll want a rough idea of how many calories you're taking in. This doesn't have to be detailed — a simple ballpark number is valuable.

MyPlate is one option (see page 185). Developed by the U.S. Department of Agriculture (USDA), this guide uses the visual of a place setting to show how many calories you're taking in.

It's simple: Fill half your plate with veggies, one-quarter with whole grains and the other quarter with a small serving of lean protein. This is a simple way to ensure you have filling, healthy meals. Apply the MyPlate concept to your meals for several days to get a general sense of your general calorie intake. If 2,000 calories a day is your goal, for example, strive for 2 cups of fruit, 2½ cups of vegetables, 6 ounces of grains, 5½ ounces of protein, and 3 cups of low-fat or fat-free dairy products each day.

Another option is to buy healthy, pre-made meals from your grocery store or meal kits that tell you exactly how many calories you're getting. This option should be temporary — just for a month — to give you a sense of your calorie intake. If you take this route, it's important to choose healthy meals that are low in sodium. (Find guidance on sodium later in this chapter.)

Next, how many calories are you burning through physical activity? You'll find detailed information on exercise in the next chapter. For now, a quick check of how much physical activity you're getting will help you see how many calories you're burning each day. You may already have a favorite tool that helps you estimate how many calories you're burning through physical activity; there are plenty of options to choose from.

One such tool is offered by the American Council on Exercise (see page 185). This

SHARON'S WEIGHT-LOSS PLAN

Sharon, 45, wants to lose weight mostly to lower her blood pressure, but also to improve her overall health. She weighs 150 pounds. She's somewhat active, getting light activity or moderate activity like a 30-minute brisk walk two or three times a week. Her basal metabolic rate — the number of calories her body needs to function — is 1,850.

Sharon checks out the American Council on Exercise tool and sees that every time she takes a 30-minute walk at a moderate pace, she's burning 112 calories. She decides to start increasing her physical activity just a little, aiming to take a 30-minute walk at a quicker pace five days each week rather than the two or three days a week she currently walks at a slower pace.

Next, Sharon looks at MyPlate to see where she can adjust her eating habits to cut back on calories. She takes a short assessment by entering her age, height, weight and activity level. She selects the calorie goal for weight loss and gets a personalized plan that shows how much food from each food group she should have in each meal to achieve her calorie goal. For now, she plans to keep her calorie count at 1,800 a day.

Now that Sharon knows how much food from each food group she should have in each meal — and how it should look on her plate — she feels confident that she has the information she needs to improve her eating habits and work toward keeping her calorie count to 1,800 a day. Add to this an increase in physical activity, and Sharon feels good about the changes she'll make and how they'll improve her health.

tool calculates many types of physical activity.

Once you know about how many calories you're taking in and how many you're burning, aim to cut 250-500 calories a day through healthier eating and more activity. Even small choices, such as replacing higher calorie foods with fruits and vegetables and moving more during the day, can help lower your weight and your blood pressure. Make sure not to drop below 1,200 calories a day, though — you need at least this many calories a day to ensure that you're getting enough nutrients.

Knowing how many calories you're taking in and how many you're burning will allow you to make small adjustments that can yield significant results in your weight, your blood pressure and your overall health.

DIAL IN ON YOUR DIET

The foods you choose for weight loss can have a significant effect on blood pressure all on their own. This is especially important when it comes to certain minerals and vitamins. Along with weight loss, the amounts of potassium and

USE ENERGY DENSITY TO GUIDE FOOD CHOICES

Energy density is the number of calories in an amount of food. By choosing foods that are low in calories, but high in volume, you can eat more and feel fuller on fewer calories. Fruits and vegetables are good choices because they tend to be low in energy density and high in volume.

Foods high in energy density include fatty foods, such as many fast foods, and foods high in sugar, such as sodas and candies. For example, a small order of fast-food fries has more than 200 calories. For the same calories, you could have a heaping helping of fresh fruits and vegetables — such as a salad made with 10 cups of spinach, 1½ cups of strawberries and a small apple. Plus, with fresh fruits and vegetables, you get a plethora of valuable nutrients — not just empty calories. These foods also take longer to eat and are filling, which helps curb your hunger.

Energy density is also important when you're snacking. If you're working on losing weight or maintaining weight loss, keep your snacks at about 100 calories. For reference, one ounce of potato chips is about 150 calories. Instead, for only 100 calories, you could snack on 3½ cups of air-popped popcorn. If you're used to a sweet ending to your meal, try fresh fruit and yogurt as a tasty, low-calorie alternative to a slice of pie.

sodium in your diet are critical to lowering blood pressure.

The power of potassium

The DASH diet emphasizes three minerals that can play a role in managing high blood pressure: potassium, calcium and magnesium. Researchers have found that a high potassium intake is associated with lower blood pressure, especially in Black people.

Potassium balances the amount of sodium in your cells. A high intake of potassium lowers blood pressure. Potassium is found in many fruits and vegetables, whole grains, legumes, dairy products and in potatoes.

A number of foods contain potassium. Good sources include: apricots, bananas, cantaloupe, cherries, dates, figs, honeydew melon, kiwi, mango, nectarine, orange, papaya, prunes and tangerines, apple juice, grapefruit juice, grape juice,

---

WEIGHT LOSS AND THE DASH DIET

To lose weight while following the DASH diet, use the serving guidelines below. This will help ensure that you're getting enough of each food group. These servings are your target if you're planning to keep your overall calories per day between 1,200 and 1,800.

Food groups	Daily servings
Whole grains	4 to 6
Vegetables	3 to 5
Fruits	4 to 5
Fat-free or low-fat milk and milk products	2 to 3
Lean meats, poultry, fish	3 to 6 or less
Nuts, seeds, legumes	3 to 4 a week
Fats and oils	1 to 3
Sweets and added sugars	1 to 3 or less a week

Source: DASH Eating Plan — Number of Food Servings by Calorie Level, National Heart, Lung, and Blood Institute, 2014.

orange juice, pineapple juice, artichokes, beans (dried), beets, broccoli, Brussels sprouts, leafy vegetables (beet greens, collard greens, spinach), kohlrabi (cooked), lentils, mushrooms, parsley, potatoes, pumpkin, soy products, squash, zucchini, cocoa powder, milk (fat-free or low-fat), peanut butter, tofu and yogurt (fat-free or low-fat).

The Institute of Medicine advises that all adult Americans eat more potassium-rich foods, such as fruits and vegetables.

Eating 8 to 10 servings a day of fruits and vegetables can help you get the recommended potassium intake of 3,500 to 5,000 mg a day. But very few adults consume this much potassium.

Some people have to be cautious about their potassium intake. If you have kidney disease, congestive heart failure or diabetes, talk to your health care team about the levels of potassium and other minerals in your diet.

Sodium's role

Sodium helps maintain the right balance of fluids in your body. It also helps transmit nerve impulses and influences the way your muscles contract and relax.

You get sodium from the foods you eat. Many foods naturally contain sodium, but about 70% of your sodium intake comes from compounds added to food during commercial processing and about 11% from meal preparation at home, added during cooking or while eating. Table salt, which is a compound of sodium and chloride, is the most common source of sodium.

Recommendations for sodium intake range from 1,200 mg a day to an upper

WHAT ABOUT POTASSIUM SUPPLEMENTS?

If you're not getting enough potassium, you may think that taking a supplement is the way to go. However, studies suggest that getting potassium from foods rather than supplements is best. Plus, potassium supplements can have serious side effects. And some blood pressure medications, such as potassium-retaining diuretics, angiotensin-converting enzyme (ACE) inhibitors, angiotensin II receptor blockers and renin inhibitors, can increase potassium levels in your blood. Take potassium supplements only if your health care team recommends them.

If you take a diuretic medication that causes your body to lose potassium, your health care team may recommend that you take a potassium supplement. Otherwise, it's best to get your potassium from the foods you eat.

limit of 2,300 mg for most healthy adults. Most Americans consume much more than that; the estimated average daily sodium intake for Americans ranges from 2,000 to 5,000 mg.

Kidneys regulate the amount of sodium in the body. When sodium levels fall, the kidneys conserve sodium. When sodium levels are high, the kidneys flush out the excess amount of sodium through urine. Genetic factors, medications, and heart, kidney, liver and lung diseases all can interfere with the body's ability to regulate sodium.

When the kidneys can't eliminate enough sodium, the mineral starts to accumulate in the blood. Because sodium attracts and holds water, blood volume increases. As a result, the heart has to work harder to move the increased volume of blood, increasing the pressure on the arteries.

Sodium sensitivity

How people's bodies react to sodium varies. Some healthy adults, including some with high blood pressure, can consume varying amounts of sodium with little or no effect on their blood pressure.

For others, too much sodium quickly leads to higher blood pressure, often triggering chronic high blood pressure. This response is referred to as sodium sensitivity or salt sensitivity.

About half of Americans with high blood pressure and a quarter of Americans with blood pressure that's at a healthy level are sodium sensitive. The condition is more common in Black people and older adults. People with diabetes or long-term kidney disease also tend to be more sensitive to high levels of sodium.

Exactly what causes sodium sensitivity isn't known, but genetic factors likely affect the way the body handles salt. This sensitivity can be passed down through families, and researchers have identified several genes associated with higher blood pressure (as well as lower blood pressure).

There's no easy way to tell if you're sodium sensitive. Some researchers have developed blood tests that can detect salt sensitivity, but more studies are needed to confirm the reliability of these tests. In addition to increasing blood pressure, sodium sensitivity can increase the risk of kidney problems and cardiovascular disease.

The controversy

Ever since the recommendation that all Americans — not just those with hyper-tension — limit sodium to control blood pressure, the issue has sparked contro-versy. While limiting sodium helps some people, when others cut back on sodium, their blood pressure decreases very little, if at all.

Critics point out that studies linking a low-sodium diet to lower blood pressure don't show improvements in actual outcomes. In other words, they say the

This guide lists foods that are low in sodium and can be eaten frequently. It complements the DASH diet.

Whole grains and starches
- Whole-grain bread, rolls and cereals with less than 200 mg of sodium in a serving
- Quick breads such as pancakes or biscuits made from home recipes that use no buttermilk and little or no salt
- Potatoes, rice and pasta
- Unsalted popcorn, pretzels, chips and crackers

Vegetables
- Fresh, unsalted frozen or low-sodium canned vegetables
- No-salt-added or low-sodium tomato juice and vegetable juice
- No-salt-added canned tomato products

Fruits
- Fresh and frozen fruit and canned fruit in juice or water

Dairy products
- Fat-free or low-fat milk, low-fat and low-sodium ricotta and cottage cheese
- Reduced-fat cheeses with less than 200 mg of sodium per ounce

Limit (2-3 times a week):
- Regular cottage cheese and aged natural cheese such as brick cheese, Monterey Jack and mild cheddar

Beverages
- Bottled water and low-sugar or no-sugar-added beverages with less than 70 mg of sodium in a serving
- Tap water (sodium content varies with the local water supply).

Limit (1-2 servings a day):
- Alcoholic beverages
- Coffee and tea
- Cocoa (made with sweetened cocoa powder)

Condiments
- No-salt-added ketchup, mustard, barbecue sauce, others

Lean meats, poultry and fish
- Fresh or frozen meat and poultry without added salt or saline
- Fresh or frozen fish and shellfish (unbreaded and not packed in brine or with added sodium)
- Water-packed canned tuna or other seafood, canned salmon with no added salt
- Egg whites

Limit (2-3 times a week):
- Canned tuna and other canned seafood packed with 50% to 60% less salt
- Reduced-sodium processed meats and cheeses
- Lobster and crab

Main dish items
- Homemade dishes and soups without added salt or canned vegetables as ingredients
- Frozen and microwave dinners that have less than 600 mg of sodium in a dinner
- Low-sodium canned broth, soups and bouillon

Nuts, seeds and legumes
- Low-sodium or no-salt-added peanut butter
- Unsalted nuts and seeds
- Dried peas, beans and lentils

Fats and oils (use sparingly)
- Oil, margarine or butter
- Salad dressings with less than 200 mg of sodium in a serving
- Mayonnaise and unsalted gravy
- Cream cheese and sour cream

Desserts and sweets (use sparingly)
- Homemade desserts, cooked pudding and box mixes with less than 200 mg sodium in a serving
- Fresh fruit, gelatin, sherbet, plain cake, meringue, ice cream and frozen yogurt
- Jams, jellies, honey, hard candy and jelly beans

studies don't prove that a low-sodium diet results in fewer deaths from conditions associated with high blood pressure such as heart disease and stroke.

Many large studies, however, show that when people consume less sodium, their blood pressure will fall and, furthermore, fewer deaths occur from heart attack and stroke. Reducing sodium intake can also lower your risk of osteoporosis, kidney disease and stomach cancer.

So while limiting sodium may benefit some people just a little, it has a major impact on the general population in preventing high blood pressure and reducing death and disability.

Even a small reduction in average blood pressure across a large population — perhaps just 5 millimeters of mercury (mm Hg) in pressure — can lead to significant positive outcomes for the overall health and well-being of that population.

The American Heart Association, the American Medical Association and various U.S. government agencies continue to monitor scientific information about sodium and blood pressure. Their positions support limiting sodium as a reasonable and safe step toward good health.

One thing that the DASH-Sodium study and other research make clear is that limiting sodium works best in the context of an overall healthy diet. For example, limiting sodium consumption in combination with losing weight and eating a healthy diet are more effective in manag-

ing high blood pressure than is limiting sodium intake alone.

Current recommendations

The Centers for Disease Control and Prevention recommends that all Americans limit sodium to less than 2,300 mg a day. That's the amount of sodium in about a teaspoon of salt. These targets are lower for infants, young children and teens.

If you have high blood pressure, your health care team may advise reducing your sodium intake even further. Making sure that you eat enough potassium-rich foods will help further to control your blood pressure levels.

Many health professionals and medical organizations, including Mayo Clinic, support a lower sodium diet. Here's why they do so:
- If you have high blood pressure, reducing sodium can lower your blood pressure. Limiting sodium, along with other lifestyle changes, may be enough to keep you from having to take medication to control your blood pressure.
- If you're taking blood pressure medication, limiting sodium can help increase the effectiveness of the drug. Even if you're taking a diuretic, it's still important to reduce sodium in your diet. (Learn more about medications in Chapter 8.)
- If you're at risk of high blood pressure, limiting sodium and making other lifestyle changes may prevent it.
- If you don't have high blood pressure, limiting sodium is still safe and reason-

able. It also may lower your risk of high blood pressure as you get older. Many health care providers say that curbing salt intake should begin in childhood, to help prevent blood pressure-related problems that may begin as early as the teen years.

PRACTICAL FOOD TIPS FOR EVERYDAY LIFE

Putting healthy eating into practice can seem overwhelming at first, but it doesn't have to be complicated. Use this advice as a guide.

At the grocery store

Success with the DASH diet starts with the foods you buy. When you're shopping, think fresh and unprocessed. These are the types of foods to focus on.

You'll find that the freshest and healthiest foods tend to be located around the perimeter of a grocery store. Try to spend most of your time in the produce section, where you can stock up on fruits and vegetables for meals and snacking. In addition, choose fresh meats instead of smoked or cured meats, such as luncheon meat, bacon, hot dogs, sausage and ham.

Use the Nutrition Facts label to your advantage. It tells you which foods are healthy and warns you about those that aren't so healthy. It can also help you compare the ingredients of similar foods and select items that are the most nutritious. See an example on the right.

FOOD LABEL EXAMPLE

This example provides a breakdown of calories, fat, carbohydrates, protein, vitamins and minerals in a single serving. Notice which components are low (5% of the Daily Value or less) and which ones are high (20% of the Daily Value or more). This food is low in saturated fat but high in added sugars. As part of a meal, the rest of the foods and beverages should have 600-700 mg of sodium or less.

Nutrition Facts	
8 servings per container	
Serving size	**2/3 cup (55g)**
Amount per serving	
Calories	**230**
	% Daily Value*
Total Fat 8g	**10%**
Saturated Fat 1g	**5%**
Trans Fat 0g	
Cholesterol 0mg	**0%**
Sodium 160mg	**7%**
Total Carbohydrate 37g	**13%**
Dietary Fiber 4g	**14%**
Total Sugars 12g	
Includes 10g Added Sugars	**20%**
Protein 3g	
Vitamin D 2mcg	10%
Calcium 260mg	20%
Iron 8mg	45%
Potassium 240mg	6%

* The % Daily Value (DV) tells you how much a nutrient in a serving of food contributes to a daily diet. 2,000 calories a day is used for general nutrition advice.

In general, any product with 5% of the Daily Value for sodium in a serving is low, while any product with 20% of the Daily Value is high. In terms of sodium, choose foods that have less than 200 mg in a serving. Keep this in mind when choosing soups, frozen dinners, sauces, condiments such as ketchup, and mixes and other instant products, as well as snacks such as potato chips, corn chips, pretzels, popcorn and crackers. Look for low-sodium versions of broths, soups and canned vegetables. Also look for low levels of fat, saturated fat and cholesterol in the foods you buy.

At restaurants

Though eating at home is generally healthiest, you can eat nutritiously away from home when you're savvy about which choices are healthiest to make.

First, it's important to be mindful of two common eating-out challenges: the urge to order more food than you need, and the impulse to eat everything on your plate. When an entree is larger than you want — which is often the case — ask if you can have the lunch portion, even if you're eating dinner. You can also request

MAKING SENSE OF SODIUM LABELING

Here's what sodium-related terms on many food labels mean:
- **Sodium-free or salt-free.** Each serving in this product contains less than 5 mg of sodium.
- **Very low sodium.** Each serving contains 35 mg of sodium or less.
- **Low sodium.** Each serving contains 140 mg of sodium or less.
- **Reduced or less sodium.** The product contains at least 25% less sodium than the regular version.
- **Lite or light in sodium.** The sodium content has been reduced by at least 50% from the regular version.
- **Unsalted or no salt added.** No salt is added during processing of a food that normally contains salt. However, some foods with these labels may still be high in sodium.

Don't be fooled — foods labeled "reduced sodium" or "light in sodium" may still contain a lot of salt. If the regular product starts out high in sodium, reducing it by 25% or 50% may make little difference. For example, a serving of regular canned chicken noodle soup may have about 844 mg of sodium per cup, while the reduced-sodium version may still have 633 mg per cup. When paired with other foods and beverages, this one meal could put you over the top for the amount of sodium you should have in one day. The bottom line? Read the labels carefully.

SPICE IT UP

It's easy to make food taste good without using salt. Try these suggestions for herbs, spices and flavorings to enhance the taste of various foods.

Meat, poultry, fish

Beef	Bay leaf, dry mustard, horseradish, marjoram, nutmeg, onion, pepper, sage, thyme
Chicken	Basil, dill, fresh tomatoes, ginger, oregano, paprika, parsley, rosemary, sage, tarragon, thyme
Fish	Bay leaf, curry powder, dill, dry mustard, lemon juice, paprika
Lamb	Cranberry, curry powder, garlic, rosemary
Pork	Cranberry, garlic, onion, oregano, pepper, sage
Veal	Bay leaf, curry powder, ginger, oregano

Vegetables

Broccoli	Lemon juice, oregano
Carrots	Cinnamon, honey, nutmeg, orange juice, rosemary, sage
Cauliflower	Nutmeg, tarragon
Corn	Chives, cumin, fresh tomatoes, green pepper, paprika, parsley
Green beans	Dill, lemon juice, nutmeg, tarragon, unsalted French dressing
Peas	Mint, onion, parsley
Potatoes	Dill, garlic, green pepper, onion, parsley, sage
Tomatoes	Basil, dill, onion, oregano, parsley, sage

Low-sodium soups

Creamed	Bay leaf, dill, paprika, peppercorns, tarragon
Vegetable	Basil, bay leaf, curry, dill, garlic, onion, oregano

Other

Popcorn	Curry, garlic powder, onion powder
Rice	Basil, cumin, curry, green pepper, oregano
Salads	Basil, dill, lemon juice, parsley, vinegar

WHAT TO LOOK FOR ON A RESTAURANT MENU

When reviewing a restaurant menu, use these tips to help you keep your eating plan on target:

Meal course	What to choose	
Appetizer	Selections with fresh vegetables, fruit or fish	
Soup	Fruit or salad in place of soup	
Salad	Lettuce or spinach salad with the dressing on the side; 1 soupspoon of dressing; olive oil with vinegar for a salad topping	
Bread	Whole-grain bread; rolls; breadsticks; bagels, plain or with a little honey, jam or jelly	
Entree	Low-fat options, such as London broil, grilled chicken breast, baked or poached fish or broiled beef or chicken kebabs; sauce on the side; lemon wedge to add flavor	
Side dish	Baked potato; boiled new potatoes; steamed vegetables; rice; fresh fruit	
Condiments	Fresh tomato, cucumber and lettuce for sandwiches; ketchup, mustard and mayonnaise only sparingly	
Dessert	Fresh fruit; poached spiced fruit; plain cake with fruit puree; sorbet or sherbet; ½ cup frozen yogurt or ice cream	

Also, keep in mind that alcohol is high in calories. Drinking too much alcohol can also raise your blood pressure. If you choose to drink alcohol, limit the amount to no more than one drink a day for women and up to two drinks a day for men. Learn more about the relationship between alcohol and high blood pressure in Chapter 7.

What to avoid

	Anything fried or breaded
	Broth- or tomato-based soups; creamed soups, pureed soups, chowders and some fruit soups
	Caesar salads and chef salads; taco salads
	Muffins; garlic toast; croissants; crackers
	Marinated items and foods with descriptions indicating higher fat content, such as prime rib of beef, veal Parmesan, stuffed shrimp, fried chicken and filet mignon with béarnaise sauce
	French fries; hash browns; twice-baked potatoes; potato chips; onion rings; mayonnaise-based salads
	Olives; pickles; sauerkraut
	All other desserts

a take-home bag when the meal is served. Or you might choose an appetizer for an entree or split a meal with a companion.

Next, look for healthy selections on the menu. Consider hidden calories, as well. These come from ingredients added to enhance the flavor, color or texture of food — for example, seasonings, sauces or dressings. And sometimes they're part of the preparation process — for example, oil or butter used in cooking. These calories add up.

At home

Several small adjustments at home can help to lower your sodium intake. These steps also can improve your overall eating habits.

Don't add salt when you cook rice, pasta and hot cereals. Remove salt from recipes whenever possible. In some recipes, you can use a no-salt product and a regular product. For example, if your recipe calls for 16 ounces of tomato sauce, try using 8 ounces of no-salt-added sauce and 8 ounces of regular sauce.

Other good choices include limiting condiments, using caution with salt substitutes, and opting for a small amount of unsalted nuts or seeds in place of a salty snack.

To make meat kosher without using salt, broil the meat in a flat pan that allows the juices to run off. To remove salt in kosher meats, place the raw meat in a large pot filled with cold water and bring the pot to a boil. Then remove the pot from the heat and drain the water. Most of the salt will drain away. You can do this twice if you need to remove all of the salt.

For people who won't eat meat if it hasn't been koshered in some way, here's another option. First, soak the nonkoshered meat in water for 30 minutes. Then, add table salt instead of koshering salt for 30 minutes versus the standard 60 minutes. Next, instead of simply

ALL SALT IS SALT

There are many different types of salt available, and some — such as sea salt — are promoted as a healthier alternative to table salt. But all types of salt have the same basic nutritional value. Sea salt and table salt, for example, contain the same amounts of sodium by weight.

The only exception to this is seasoned salt. Seasoned salt is salt mixed with herbs and spices. Garlic salt, onion salt and celery salt are other examples. Seasoned salt is still high in sodium but generally has slightly less sodium than does table salt.

rinsing the meat, soak it again for 30 minutes. Soak it twice if needed.

It will take your taste buds several weeks to months to adjust to the taste of food prepared with less salt. But if you stick with it, highly salted food will soon begin to taste unpleasant. It's not much different from switching from whole milk to skim milk. When you first make this change, skim milk may lack taste and seem watered down. But over time whole milk products eventually often taste too thick and rich.

PUTTING IT IN PERSPECTIVE

Remember that eating well isn't an all-or-nothing proposition. Perfection isn't the goal — being persistent in your pursuit of healthy eating is what's most important. Over time, these approaches will become habits that will help you manage your blood pressure, improve your health, control your weight and feel better about yourself.

Movement is medicine

6

Physical activity, along with healthy eating, is vital for reducing and controlling blood pressure. Regular activity can lower systolic and diastolic blood pressure by about the same amount as many blood pressure medications.

One reason why high blood pressure is so common may be that people aren't active enough. Modern conveniences and a shortage of free time have caused Americans to become increasingly sedentary.

According to a Centers for Disease Control and Prevention survey, fewer than 1 in 4 of American adults get the amount of aerobic activity and strength training recommended in the Department of Health and Human Services' Physical Activity Guidelines for Americans. Almost half of American adults don't get enough of either type.

Using physical activity to help lower blood pressure doesn't mean spending long hours at the gym. It's not necessary to live by the motto "No pain, no gain," pushing yourself to the limits of your endurance. On the contrary, it's enough that you remain committed and make every effort to be physically active on a daily basis.

Moderate activity is good for your heart and overall health. Movement is medicine, and any amount helps. A key element to receiving these benefits, however, is that you exercise regularly.

One way to do this is to find activities that you enjoy. Remember: Anything that gets you moving counts, whether it's a brisk walk, swimming or any other activity you like to do.

BENEFITS OF REGULAR ACTIVITY

Physical activity is important for controlling blood pressure because it makes the heart stronger and more efficient. With greater strength, the heart can pump more blood with less effort. And the better the heart can pump blood, the less force is exerted on the arteries.

Regular physical activity can lower blood pressure by as much as 4 to 12 millimeters of mercury (mm Hg) diastolic and 3 to 6 mm Hg systolic. If you're at risk of high blood pressure, that's low enough to keep the condition from ever developing. If you have high blood pressure, lowering it slightly may be enough to prevent you from having to take medication to control it. If you're taking medication, this is enough to help it lower your blood pressure more effectively.

Being physically active can improve health in many ways. In addition to helping control blood pressure, regular physical activity reduces the risk of heart attack, high cholesterol, diabetes, osteoporosis and 13 different types of cancer. It improves energy, boosts mood, improves sleep and helps with stress and anxiety.

In addition, regular activity helps with weight loss. When you gain weight, blood pressure often increases. And when you lose weight, blood pressure often goes down. The most successful method of losing weight includes getting regular, moderate physical activity most days of the week.

Activity vs. intensity

For many years, the belief was that you had to exercise vigorously to be physically fit and to improve health. As a result, people developed an all-or-nothing attitude toward exercise. And this led to a high dropout rate.

But studies show that light activity is also good for your blood pressure and overall health — and it's better than doing nothing at all. For most healthy adults, the Department of Health and Human Services recommends these exercise guidelines:

Aerobic activity

Get at least 150 minutes a week of moderate aerobic activity or 75 minutes a week of vigorous aerobic activity. Moderate activity should be "moderately intense," which means that breathing quickens and the heart beats a little faster. You can gauge this effort as being somewhere between 11 and 14 on the perceived exertion scale (see "Perceived exertion scale" on page 95). You can also do a combination of moderate and vigorous activity. The guidelines suggest spreading out this exercise over the course of a week. The more activity, the greater the health benefits.

Strength training

Do strength training exercises at least twice a week. Focus on the major muscle groups in your arms, legs and core.

The guidelines don't offer a set amount of time for each strength training session.

In addition to common recreational activities, such as walking, bicycling and dancing, the guidelines promote routine activities such as mowing the lawn, gardening, washing the car, cleaning the house and climbing stairs. The more you move about during the day, the less you sit, and the more calories you burn during

---

ARE YOU FIT?

1. Do you have enough energy to enjoy the leisure activities you like to do?
    - ☐ Rarely or never (1 point)
    - ☐ Sometimes (2 points)
    - ☐ Always or most of the time (3 points)

2. Do you have enough stamina and strength to carry out the daily tasks of your life?
    - ☐ Rarely or never (1 point)
    - ☐ Sometimes (2 points)
    - ☐ Always or most of the time (3 points)

3. Can you walk a mile without feeling winded or fatigued?
    - ☐ No (1 point)
    - ☐ Sometimes (2 points)
    - ☐ Yes (3 points)

4. Can you climb two flights of stairs without feeling winded or fatigued?
    - ☐ No (1 point)
    - ☐ Sometimes (2 points)
    - ☐ Yes (3 points)

5. Are you flexible enough to touch your toes?
    - ☐ No (1 point)
    - ☐ Sometimes (2 points)
    - ☐ Yes (3 points)

the day through the activities of daily life, such as tapping your foot (known as nonexercise activity thermogenesis, or NEAT), washing clothes and sweeping the floor, the more health benefits you'll gain.

An activity doesn't have to be condensed into one block of time in your busy schedule. The cumulative effect of physical activity throughout the day is what matters. For example, taking a short bike ride in the morning, using the stairs instead of the elevator at work, and spending time working in your flower beds in the afternoon can add up, equaling a single workout session at the gym.

6. Can you carry on a conversation while doing light to moderately intense activities, such as brisk walking?
   ☐ No (1 point)
   ☐ Sometimes (2 points)
   ☐ Yes (3 points)

7. About how many days a week do you spend doing at least 30 minutes of moderately vigorous activity, such as walking briskly or raking leaves?
   ☐ Zero to two days (1 point)
   ☐ Three to four days (2 points)
   ☐ Five to seven days (3 points)

»» How did you score?

To the right of the answer you chose is a point value — 1, 2 or 3 points. Add up the points from your answers for your total score.

A: If your total score was 18 to 21 points, congratulations! You're well on your way to overall fitness.

B: If your score was 13 to 17 points, you're on the right track, but your activity level could use a little boost.

C: If your score was 7 to 12 points, it's time to put getting in shape at the top of your to-do list.

That said, don't discount the benefits of vigorous exercise. The guidelines are meant to complement — not replace — previous advice promoting high-intensity interval training. More vigorous activity can bring greater health benefits. For example, interval training — short, 30-second bouts of intense exercise performed during your exercise session — has been shown to be particularly beneficial in improving fitness in an effective and efficient manner. This is true even for people with a history of heart disease.

The main goal is to take part in some type of physical activity for 30 to 60 minutes most days of the week.

WHAT KIND OF ACTIVITY?

Physical fitness typically involves three components: aerobic activity to improve your heart and lung capacity (cardiovas-cular health), exercises that improve flexibility in your joints and muscles, and strengthening exercises to build and maintain bone and muscle mass.

An activity is aerobic when it places added demands on your heart, lungs and muscles, increasing your body's ability to use oxygen. As a result, you can produce more energy and won't tire as quickly. Aerobic activity increases your endurance and stamina, which helps you do the things you want to do. Cleaning house, playing golf and swimming laps all are aerobic activities if they require a fairly light to somewhat hard effort. Other forms of aerobic activity include:

Walking

Walking appeals to many people because it doesn't require special athletic skills or instruction. It's convenient and inexpen-sive, and you can vary the route to keep it

---

PHYSICAL ACTIVITY VS. EXERCISE

The terms *physical activity* and *exercise* are closely related — and often overlap — but there's a difference. Physical activity refers to any body movement that burns calories, such as raking leaves or taking the dog for a walk. Exercise is a more structured form of physical activity. It generally involves repetitive movements that strengthen or develop a part of the body and improve cardiovascular fitness. Exercise includes walking, swimming and biking.

Therefore, exercise is a form of physical activity, but not all physical activity fits the definition of exercise. Either way, many health benefits may be gained through regular physical activity, even if it's not in a structured, repetitive form.

PERCEIVED EXERTION SCALE

Exercise intensity reflects the amount of oxygen the body uses. The perceived exertion scale estimates exercise intensity. Perceived exertion is the total amount of effort and stress you feel during activity, including heart rate, breathing rate, perspiration and muscle fatigue.

The scale ranges from 6, representing the body at rest, to 20, representing maximum effort. Moderate activity ranges from 11 to 14. You can gauge your perceived effort during exercise. For example, adjust a brisk beach walk to what you perceive as about an 11 on the exertion scale in order to maintain a moderate pace.

Any physical activity is helpful, but to get the most benefit, activity should be moderately intense, which means that your breathing quickens and you feel your heart beat a little faster.

6	10	14	18
7 - Very, very light	11 - Fairly light	15 - Hard	19 - Very, very hard
8	12	16	20
9 - Very light	13 - Somewhat hard	17 - Very hard	

© Borg G. Borg Rating of Perceived Exertion Scale. 1998.

Your perception of exercise intensity is more important than your absolute level of exertion. For example, brisk walking at 3 to 4 mph may feel like light exercise to a physically fit person but like strenuous exercise to someone who's not in shape. Both individuals will benefit from what they perceive as moderate exercise, although they'll walk at a different pace.

interesting. You can enjoy it alone or with friends. It's also low impact, so if you have arthritis in your hips, knees or ankles, it usually won't cause a flare-up in your symptoms.

When walking, wear good shoes that give your feet support and traction. If you've been inactive and you're out of shape, start at a very light pace for five to 10 minutes. Gradually increase the intensity and duration of your walks, with a goal of walking 30 to 60 minutes each time.

Jogging

Jogging is an excellent form of aerobic exercise because it provides a good workout for your heart, lungs and muscles in a relatively brief period of time.

At the same time, jogging doesn't have to be strenuous to have a positive effect. You can go at your own pace. Like walking, jogging doesn't require a lot of equipment — you just need a good pair of athletic shoes.

Be advised, however, that jogging requires some cardiovascular conditioning and muscle strengthening before you start. If you haven't been active for several months, start by walking. When you can walk 2 miles in 30 minutes comfortably, you're ready to try alternating jogging with walking. Gradually increase the amount of time you spend jogging and decrease the amount of time you spend walking.

To minimize your risk of injury and muscle and joint discomfort, don't jog more than three or four times a week and try to jog on alternate days. If you have arthritis, this form of exercise can contribute to pain or discomfort in your knees, hips or ankles.

HOW DO I FIND THE TIME TO EXERCISE?

Lack of time seems to be a common obstacle to exercise. But often, it's priorities rather than time that's the real issue. Being more physically active may mean spending less time doing something else — perhaps a half hour less spent online or watching TV. Here are some ways to fit exercise into your daily schedule.

- Walk for 10 minutes over your lunch hour or get up a few minutes earlier in the morning and go for a short walk. Or take a walk with your family after dinner in the evening.
- Get up from your desk to stretch and walk around during your workday.
- Instead of looking for shortcuts from one location to another, look for ways to add an extra minute or two of walking.
- Schedule time with a friend to do physical activities together on a regular basis

ACTIVITY GUIDE

Activity	Calories burned per hour for a 150-pound adult
Basketball (playing a game)	544
Basketball (shooting baskets)	306
Bicycling	510
Dancing	530
Gardening	258
Lawn mowing (push mower)	374
Playing touch football	544
Playing volleyball	272
Raking leaves	258
Running (13 minutes per mile)	408
Shoveling snow (by hand, moderate effort)	360
Stair climbing (slow pace)	272
Swimming laps (freestyle, front crawl, slow, light or moderate effort)	394
Walking (moderate pace on a level, firm surface)	238
Walking (very, very brisk pace on a level, firm surface)	476
Washing and waxing a car	136
Washing windows and floors	238
Water aerobics	374
Wheeling self in wheelchair (firm, flat surface, 2 mph)	224

Based on © Ainsworth BE, et al. 2011 compendium of physical activities: A second update of codes and MET values. Medicine & Science in Sports & Exercise. 2011;43:1575

Bicycling

Like walking, bicycling is a good choice if you're starting a regular exercise program. This low-impact activity is great for people with joint problems such as arthritis. And bicycling offers a change of scenery with each session. Start slowly and build up to about 30 minutes or more three to six times a week.

You may be tempted to challenge yourself by setting the gears to make pedaling hard, producing a strain resembling that of a hard run. This gives you muscle fatigue but often doesn't work your heart and lungs effectively. A cadence of 80 to 100 revolutions per minute (RPMs) is best.

Are you worried about traffic with bicycling or you don't care to chance the outdoors? A stationary bike is a good choice. These machines can be upright or reclining (recumbent), and one type is not inherently better than the other — the choice is yours.

Stationary bikes give you mainly a lower body workout, but some have moving handlebars that increase the demands on your heart and lungs.

If you have knee problems, adjust the resistance to a low setting, and make sure that the seat height is appropriate for you. Your knee should be bent at a slight angle — just short of being totally straight.

HOW DO I KNOW IF I'M FIT ENOUGH TO EXERCISE?

Fitness is an individual quality that's influenced by age, sex, genetic makeup, eating habits, regular activity level and the presence of a chronic health condition. You're fit if you can:

- Carry out daily tasks without getting overly tired and still have energy to enjoy leisurely pursuits.
- Walk a mile or climb a few flights of stairs without becoming winded or feeling heaviness or fatigue in your legs.
- Carry on a brief conversation using short sentences during moderate exercise such as brisk walking.

If you're out of shape, you:

- Feel tired much of the time.
- Fatigue quickly.
- Can't keep up with others your age.
- Avoid certain activities because you know you'll soon tire.

Exercise machines

Each of the six basic exercise machines offers specific fitness benefits to help you build aerobic capacity. In addition to the stationary bicycles mentioned previously, there are rowing machines, treadmills, stair climbers, cross-country machines and elliptical machines.

In general, you get what you pay for when you purchase an exercise machine. Look at the warranty — it's usually a sign of quality. Make sure the device is solidly built, with no exposed cables or chains, and that it operates smoothly. Avoid equipment with spring-operated components.

You can consult an expert at a local gym or fitness club to get recommendations. You may be able to try out different models.

Swimming and water exercise

Swimming is an excellent form of cardiovascular exercise because it conditions your heart and lungs, as well as all the muscles in your body. It's also gentle on your joints. If you have arthritis or another joint disease, swimming is a good way to increase aerobic activity. Try to swim for 30 minutes several times each week.

If lap swimming isn't your style, consider water aerobics or just walking in a pool. Water also has greater resistance than air, which means walking in water requires more effort and ultimately burns more calories than walking on land. The water's buoyancy prevents falls, unloads your joints and may aid circulation in people with blood flow problems in their lower extremities.

HOW MUCH ACTIVITY?

No matter what activity you choose to do, your muscles and joints need time to get accustomed to different demands. If you've been inactive, start with five- or 10-minute periods of activity at a time and build up gradually in one-minute increments. At first, try to exercise three times a week. Add more days after you've gotten used to exercise. Increasing the time gradually reduces the risk of injury and discomfort.

EXERCISE AND YOUR BLOOD PRESSURE

To get a true picture of your blood pressure level when you're monitoring it at home, measure it before you exercise instead of afterward. That's because your blood pressure may fall to a temporarily low level for a certain amount of time after exercising.

Your goal is to be as active as you can each day. At a minimum, work toward getting at least 150 minutes of moderate aerobic activity a week. (See "Activity guide" on page 97.) For moderately intense activities, that equals about 30 minutes. Lighter activities require more time; vigorous activities require less time.

The more you weigh, the less time it takes to burn calories. Likewise, the less you weigh, the more time it takes to burn calories. If you use 30 minutes as your guide, you'll be close to getting the minimum amount of activity you need.

Remember, if it's hard to carve out 30 minutes for physical activity, break it up throughout the day. Look for any opportunity to include more activity within your regular routine.

The basic fitness plan that follows outlines how to start an activity program, how to add time or distance as your fitness improves and how to add strength training to round out your overall fitness.

Building a basic fitness plan

Anyone can become more physically active. It's never too late to start, regardless of your age, weight or experience. But taking those first steps to being more active sometimes isn't as easy as it may seem.

Many people start to exercise but don't stick with it, often because they try to do too much too soon. An all-or-nothing mentality is a recipe for discouragement,

not to mention possible injury. Tailor your expectations to your fitness level, health concerns, available time and motivation.

If you have a chronic health condition or are at significant risk of cardiovascular disease, special precautions may apply. Check with your health care team before starting an exercise program if you have cardiovascular or lung disease, diabetes, arthritis, kidney disease or any condition requiring medical care.

It's also important to check with your health care team if you have symptoms of heart, lung or other serious disease. These symptoms include:
- Pain or discomfort in your chest, neck, jaw or arms during physical activity.
- Dizziness or fainting with exercise or exertion.
- Shortness of breath with mild exertion, at rest or when lying down or going to bed.
- Ankle swelling, especially at night.
- A rapid or pronounced heartbeat.
- A heart murmur that your health care team has previously diagnosed.
- Lower leg pain when you walk, which goes away with rest.

Finally, talk with your health care team before engaging in vigorous physical activity if two or more of the following apply:
- You're a man older than age 45 or a woman older than age 55.
- You have a family history of heart-related problems before age 55 in men and age 65 in women.
- You smoke or quit smoking in the past six months.

- You're overweight or obese.
- You haven't exercised for at least 30 minutes, three days a week for three months or more.
- You have high blood pressure or high cholesterol.
- You have prediabetes.

If you take medication, ask your health care team whether physical activity will change how the medication works. Drugs for diabetes and cardiovascular disease may cause dehydration, impaired balance and blurred vision. Some medications also can affect the way your body reacts to exercise.

Set your goals

Goal setting is a way to work toward meeting your expectations, and it can help you to stay motivated. When you set goals, consider your fitness level, any health concerns, available time and motivation.

Try setting simple goals that are achievable in a reasonably short amount of time. It's easy to get frustrated and give up on goals that are too ambitious or that take too long to achieve.

Often, overall goals (outcome goals) can be met through a series of smaller goals (process goals) that build on each other.

For example, if you have high blood pressure, one of your outcome goals should be to reach a target blood pressure level set by you and your health care team. Another might be to lose weight.

Your outcome goals may be:
- I will lower my systolic blood pressure by 4 mm Hg and my diastolic pressure by 2 mm Hg within six months.
- I will lose 5 pounds in six months.

You can plan to achieve these outcomes with a series of process goals. Here are some examples:
- I will avoid the elevator at work and use the stairs.
- I will be active at least 15 minutes every afternoon doing gardening, yard work or housework.
- I will walk for 30 to 60 minutes three days a week.
- I will do strengthening exercises two days a week.
- I will stretch before and after all exercise.

Note that process goals generally involve specific actions. Write down all your goals. Always be prepared to change or adjust them to suit your needs or to set new goals. Within a few days, if your goals aren't working for you, try something new and keep experimenting until you find what works for you.

Keep in mind that each experiment you try is a step you're taking toward achieving your goals and reaching your wellness vision. Whether it's successful or not, each experiment can help you learn about yourself and give you new ideas to try.

Outcome goals help you focus on the desired result and keep you moving forward. People who can stay physically active for six months usually end up making it a habit.

Calf stretch

Stand an arm's length from the wall. Lean into the wall. Place one leg forward with knee bent. Keep other leg back with your knee straight and your heel down. Keeping back straight, move hips toward the wall until you feel a stretch. Hold for 30 seconds. Relax. Repeat with the other leg.

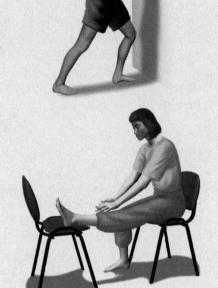

Hamstring stretch

Sit securely on a low table or a chair with one leg propped on another chair. Without bending your knee, keep your back straight and lean forward until you feel a gentle pull at the back of your thigh. Hold the position for 30 seconds. Relax. Repeat with the other leg. (You can also do this exercise sitting on the floor with one leg out front and the other bent backward.)

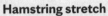

Lower back stretch

Lie on a flat surface, such as the floor or a table, with your knees bent and feet flat on the surface. Grasp one knee and pull toward your shoulders. Stop when you feel a stretch in your lower back. Hold for 30 seconds. Relax. Repeat with the other leg.

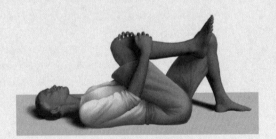

Assemble your clothing and equipment

Your choice of exercise clothing depends on your activity and the weather or location where you exercise. In general, choose comfortable, nonrestrictive items that help you feel safe, supported and dry. It's better to underdress than to overdress because exercise generates body heat.

Today's activewear often uses high-tech performance fabrics that draw sweat away from the skin to the outer surface of the garment, where it evaporates quickly. These fabrics won't stop you from sweating, but they'll keep your skin drier.

Athletic footwear may be the single most important exercise item because for many activities, your feet take the biggest beating. Shoes should be the proper width, with cushioning or shock absorption, arch support, some flexibility and wiggle room for your toes.

Good walking shoes are stable from side to side and have a rocker sole design that encourages the foot to roll and push off the toes in a natural walking motion. It's fine to wear running shoes if your primary activity is walking, as long as your feet feel comfortable and supported.

If you mostly jog or run, steer clear of shoes designed for walking. Your feet sustain a more forceful impact when you run. The shoes should provide extra cushioning to protect bones and joints.

If you plan to bicycle, look for a helmet that's well ventilated and easy to use with snug straps. If you have trouble adjusting the helmet to fit your head, you're less likely to use it. A helmet should stay in place when pushed upward from the front and shouldn't tilt in any direction or slide. Try the helmet on before you buy it.

Adjust your bicycle for your height and arm length. When you're seated with your foot on the pedal nearest the ground, your leg should be almost fully extended. You should be able to reach the handlebars and work the brakes and shift while keeping your eyes on the road.

Take time to stretch

Flexibility is the ability to move your joints through their full range of motion. You increase or maintain flexibility by regularly stretching your muscles, particularly before and after exercise. Stretching helps improve your coordination and posture, relieves stress and reduces your risk of injury.

Stretching for five to 10 minutes before an activity helps prepare your body for aerobic exercise. Be sure to warm up briefly before you stretch because stretching a cold muscle can strain the tissue. Find simple stretches on page 102.

If you have time to stretch only once during a workout, it's often helpful to warm up with the activity you'll be doing at a low level for five to 10 minutes. Stretching after your activity session, when muscles are warmed up, is often helpful to improve overall flexibility in your muscles and joints and helps prevent muscle soreness.

SIMPLE STRENGTHENING EXERCISES

Wall push-up
Face the wall and stand far enough away that you can place your palms on the wall with your elbows slightly bent. Slowly bend your elbows and lean toward the wall, supporting your weight with your arms. Straighten your arms and return to a standing position. This strengthens muscles in your arms and chest.

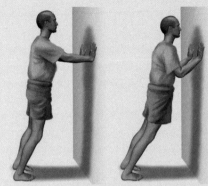

Step-up
Get a small step stool or stand in front of your stairs. Pushing primarily through your lead foot, lift your body up onto the step. Then step backward to the starting position. When you're doing step-ups, keep your back straight and your abdominal muscles nice and tight. Make sure your foot is planted entirely on the step. It's fine to start with a low step height, as well. For this exercise, your form is more important than the step height. When you step up, alternate your lead foot each time.

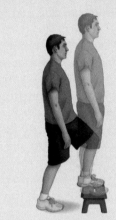

Arm curl
Stand with your feet shoulder width apart. For resistance, hold a partially filled half-gallon milk jug. Flex your elbow until your hand reaches shoulder height. Hold, then lower your arm slowly. This tones your biceps and helps in carrying and lifting. Remember to keep your wrist rigid while lifting — don't bend or curl your wrist.

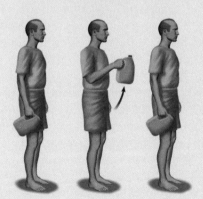

Focus on aerobic fitness

On most days, spend at least 30 minutes doing an activity such as walking, jogging, biking and swimming. This will develop your aerobic capacity, which means your heart, lungs and blood vessels can efficiently transport large amounts of oxygen throughout your body. As a result, you can produce more energy and won't fatigue as quickly. You'll also burn more calories, control your appetite, increase your stamina and sleep better at night.

Depending on your level of fitness, aerobic activity should be fairly light to somewhat hard. If you have been inactive and are out of shape, begin with just three to five minutes at a very light pace. Then gradually increase your time by one to three minutes per session and increase your pace. Many people start a program with frenzied zeal and then quit when their muscles and joints become sore or injured.

After you've been active for a while and feel you're ready, gradually pick up the pace or increase the time you spend doing your activity by a few minutes each day. For example, if you've been exercising for 30 minutes most days of the week, try aiming for 45 to 60 minutes.

When doing aerobic activities, keep these suggestions in mind:

Mix your activities

Doing the same thing all the time makes it more likely that you'll get bored and lose interest in your program. Think of more uncommon aerobic activities, such as canoeing, ballroom dancing or water exercise. In addition, try to alternate among activities that emphasize lower and upper body fitness. Participating in more than one activity (cross-training) reduces your chance of overusing or straining a muscle or joint while underusing another.

Be flexible

On days when you're overly tired or not feeling well, don't force yourself to exercise. Be willing to take a short break from your program. And as soon as you're able, get back on track with an activity you enjoy.

Listen to your body

Start slowly and give your body a chance to get used to increased activity. Stretching is key to staying flexible and maintaining a range of motion in your muscles and joints. Muscle soreness after exercise is common, especially if it's new activity, but pain during exercise may send a different signal. Be aware of signs of overexertion or stress. (See "Avoiding injury" on page 109.)

Build strength

At least twice a week, spend 20 to 30 minutes doing exercises that help build the strength and endurance of your muscles. Strength training is also called resistance training or weight training. This doesn't mean you'll bulk up. The increased lean muscle mass from these exercises simply provides you with a bigger "engine" to burn calories, helps you control your weight, and makes it easier to perform the activities of daily living.

Strength training is especially important as you get older because your muscle mass diminishes with age. Having greater muscle strength also makes aerobic activity easier. In addition, stronger muscles, tendons and ligaments around your joints help protect you from falls and fractures and reduce your risk of injury.

You build strength when your muscles push or pull against an opposing force, such as weight or gravity. The resistance can be achieved in many ways — moving or pushing against your own body weight, pulling on an elastic band or lifting weighted objects such as barbells and dumbbells.

The amount of weight or resistance you need to build muscle depends on your current strength. Choose a resistance that makes you feel as though you're working at a somewhat hard level.

As you become stronger, you can increase the weight or resistance or the number of repetitions. See "Guidelines for strength training" below.

Get instruction if you've never used strength training equipment before. You'll want to learn proper technique,

GUIDELINES FOR STRENGTH TRAINING

- Complete all movements slowly and with control. If you're unable to maintain good form and posture, decrease the weight or number of repetitions.
- If you have high blood pressure, talk to your health care team before lifting heavy weights. The strain of lifting can cause a sharp increase in your blood pressure. This could possibly be dangerous if your high blood pressure is uncontrolled.
- Breathe normally and freely, exhaling as you lift a weight and inhaling as you lower it. Holding your breath during lifting can raise your blood pressure dramatically.
- Stop exercising immediately if you feel any pain.
- Try to stretch your muscles before and after your workout. When stretching beforehand, warm up first by walking.
- It's normal to experience mild muscle soreness for a few days after starting strength training. Always allow at least one day in between strength training sessions so that your muscles can rest.

safety precautions and different kinds of exercises to do with the equipment.

You can make your own weights by filling old socks with beans or pennies, or partially filling a half-gallon milk jug with water or sand. You also can buy used weights by the pound at some athletic equipment stores. A resistance band can help you work major muscle groups.

Start with a weight that you can lift about 12 to 15 times before tiring your muscles. If you're a beginner, you may find that you're able to lift only 1 or 2 pounds in a set. That's OK. The weight should be heavy enough to tire your muscles but not cause pain.

If you start with too much resistance or too many repetitions, you may damage muscles and joints. Wait for your body to become accustomed to the exercise before gradually increasing intensity.

Staying motivated

It will likely take several months to achieve a desirable level of fitness. Your goal from then on is to maintain that level of physical fitness. Take these steps to keep yourself motivated:

Track your progress

Measure your progress with an online tracker or a written log or diary. Seeing on paper how your fitness has improved can help keep you motivated to continue and do more.

Adapt your activities

As you become more fit, fine-tune the intensity and duration of your activities to better suit your interests and lifestyle.

Try new activities

Keep your workouts enjoyable by including different and more challenging activities. Also look for ways to include family members and friends in your physical activities.

Here's one more reason to stay active: Although the generally recommended amount of exercise can make positive changes, when you stop exercising, blood pressure typically returns to its prior level.

Exercise and weight control

When combined with proper nutrition, regular physical activity does what hundreds of fad diets promise but never seem to deliver: Regular physical activity helps you lose weight and keep it off. Simply put, exercise burns calories. And when you burn more calories than you take in, you can reduce your body fat.

Here's a recap of how it works: Your body requires a certain amount of energy to maintain the functions you need to sustain life. That's your basal metabolic rate. When you exercise, your body works harder and needs more fuel (calories) to function. Even after you stop exercising, your body continues to burn calories at a modestly increased rate for a few hours.

The more intensely you exercise, the more calories you burn.

According to the Department of Health and Human Services, people trying to lose weight should aim for 300 minutes of moderately intense exercise a week or 150 minutes a week of vigorous physical activity. Moderately intense exercise includes activities such as brisk walking, biking and swimming. If you can't reach this goal right away, that's OK. Work toward it.

Physical activity helps you not only to lose weight but also to keep it off. So don't stop exercising just because you've lost a few pounds. People who are at a healthy weight need just as much physical activity as those who are trying to reach a healthy weight. Weight control combined with regular exercise reduces the risk of high blood pressure, even if you're already at a higher risk.

Avoiding injury

Occasional soreness, stiffness or minor aches and pains are to be expected with physical activity. Muscle soreness for a day or two after exercise is normal, especially if you have been inactive or are trying a new activity.

Most injuries that occur during physical activity stem from the "terrible toos" — too much, too hard, too fast, too soon,

---

HOW CAN I EXERCISE WHEN I HAVE PAINFUL ARTHRITIS IN BOTH OF MY KNEES?

For many people with pain problems, exercise can be helpful. In the case of arthritis, proper exercise can help you better maintain joint mobility.

Here are several ways to stay active:
- Try water exercises. The buoyancy of water takes the weight off your joints. You can swim laps on your own, or try a water aerobics class.
- Walk or use a stationary or recumbent bicycle. These are low-impact activities that don't put a lot of pressure on your knees.
- Consider joining a basic yoga or tai chi class to increase strength and flexibility in your joints.
- See a physical therapist who can offer recommendations on the best type of exercises for you and teach you how to do them properly to avoid injury and further pain. For example, nonpainful ways of strengthening the muscles of the knee joint can help unload the pressure on the cushioning cartilage and lessen pain.

too long. If you feel pain during exercise, this can be a warning sign of impending injury. Gasping for breath and having sore joints are other signals to slow down. Remember: If what you're doing hurts, then you're likely overdoing it. Consider reducing the intensity of the exercise or trying a different activity.

Another common cause of aches and pains is doing the same activities over and over without variation. This can lead to overuse injuries, caused by repeated stress on a particular part of your body.

Take these steps to reduce your risk of injury from exercise:

Drink plenty of water

Exercise causes you to lose some of the fluid in your body that helps maintain your normal body temperature and cool working muscles. Help replenish those fluids by drinking water before, during and after activity.

Warm up and cool down

Stretching before a workout prepares your body for physical activity. Stretching afterward helps improve your flexibility. Warm up briefly before stretching cold muscles to avoid muscle strains.

Be active regularly

In general, the less fit you are, the greater your chance of getting injured. Avoid being a weekend warrior, getting most of your activity on two days of the week. Going back and forth between intense workouts and inactivity increases your risk of injury.

Follow the 10% rule

If you want to make your exercise more intense, limit increases to about 10%. For example, if you swim laps for 30 minutes this week, plan to increase your workout to 33 minutes the next week, and so forth.

Avoid abrupt change of direction

A controlled, continuous activity, such as walking or cycling, generally carries less risk of a muscle pull or other injury than do activities in which you change direction quickly and frequently, such as basketball or tennis.

Don't compete

Unless you thrive on competition, avoid the physical and emotional intensity that often accompanies competitive sports. A less stressful environment typically allows you to stay in control of your body and not overextend yourself, which can result in harm or injury.

Let food digest

Wait three to four hours after eating a large meal before being physically active. Digestion directs blood toward your digestive system and away from your heart.

Tailor your activity to the environment

When it's hot and humid outside, reduce your speed and distance. Or exercise early in the morning or late in the evening when it's cooler. Avoid activity near heavy traffic. Breathing carbon monoxide given off by automobiles reduces the oxygen supply to your heart.

Know the warning signs

Seek immediate care if you experience any of these signs and symptoms:
- Tightness in your chest.
- Severe shortness of breath.
- Fast, irregular heartbeats (palpitations).
- Chest pain or pain in your arms or jaw, often on the left side.
- Dizziness, faintness or feeling sick to your stomach.

What about illness?

If you feel tired or achy, should you exercise? The answer may depend on your illness. If you have a cold, moderate exercise won't make it worse or prolong it. But if you have an infection and a fever, exercising increases the risk of dehydration, dangerously high body temperature and even heart failure.

One common guideline for determining whether or not you should exercise is to do a "neck check." If your signs and symptoms are above the neck — a stuffy or runny nose, sneezing or a sore throat — then moderate exercise is generally safe, although with caution. If you start feeling miserable, stop exercising.

It's best to avoid intense activity if your signs and symptoms are below the neck. These include muscle aches, hacking cough, fever, extreme fatigue, vomiting, diarrhea, chills and swollen lymph glands.

KEY POINTS

- Regular physical activity usually can reduce blood pressure by 4 to 9 mm Hg.
- Exercising regularly is more important than the intensity of exercise.
- Get at least 150 minutes of moderate physical activity, 75 minutes of vigorous physical activity or a combination of the two each week.
- Both aerobic activity and strength training can lower blood pressure. Include both in your exercise program.
- If time for exercise is a problem, look for ways to include more activity in your daily routine.

GET MORE THAN JUST EXERCISE

Do you generally get up to stretch your legs and move around after you've been seated for an hour while at work or at play? If you said no, consider changing your habits. Moving more throughout your day — in addition to getting structured exercise — is important for your health.

Cutting back on the time you spend sitting is a step in the right direction. Overwhelming research finds that too much sedentary time, which includes time spent sitting while watching TV, working on a computer or traveling in an automobile, can contribute to many health problems. This is true even for people who are very active and fit.

Sitting is something that most people have to do from time to time out of necessity. The trick is to balance your sitting time with periods of movement, through physical activity and structured exercise. When you move around or even just stand, the largest muscles of your body are actively working to keep you upright and moving, and sucking up fats and sugar from your bloodstream.

Aim for five to 10 minutes of low-intensity physical activity each hour and try to limit the amount of time you sit. Getting a drink, going to the bathroom and simply walking to a meeting are great ways to break up prolonged sedentary time. If you have a desk job or regularly sit at work, think of creative ways to cut down on the amount of time you spend sitting. Consider setting a reminder in your email calendar or on your smartphone to prompt you to get up and move.

And there are plenty of other ways to sit less throughout the day:
- Limit your TV, computer and video game use. Set a timer if you need to.
- Stand while talking on the phone.
- Put a notepad on a bookcase, so you can take notes without sitting.
- Raise your desk surface so that you can stand while you work.
- When you need to meet with someone (for work or volunteer activities), suggest a walking meeting.
- Do jumping jacks, crunches or stretches while you watch TV.

7

Avoid tobacco, limit alcohol

While smoking has not been proved to cause high blood pressure, each cigarette you smoke increases your blood pressure for a short time and raises your risk of heart attack and stroke. These are clear warnings about the dangers of smoking.

Tobacco contains a highly addictive drug called nicotine. Nicotine is the substance that makes it so difficult to stop smoking, even if you want to. It's also what causes your blood pressure to increase shortly after you take the first puff.

Like many other chemicals in tobacco smoke, nicotine is picked up by tiny blood vessels in the lungs and carried through the bloodstream. It takes only a few seconds for the drug to reach the brain. The brain reacts to nicotine by telling the adrenal glands to release epinephrine (adrenaline). This powerful hormone

narrows the blood vessels, forcing the heart to pump harder under higher pressure. The carbon monoxide in tobacco smoke replaces some of the oxygen in the blood. When the body doesn't get all the oxygen it needs, the heart and lungs have to work even harder.

After smoking just one cigarette, blood pressure can increase by about 20 millimeters of mercury (mm Hg) and stay at this higher level for about 15 minutes after you finish smoking. As the effects of smoking wear off, blood pressure gradually decreases. However, if you smoke regularly, blood pressure will stay higher throughout the day. If you smoke, regularly measure your blood pressure at home. Let your health care team know if your home readings are higher than those during your checkups.

Another important note: Nicotine adds to caffeine's effect on blood pressure.

Consuming caffeinated coffee, tea and soft drinks while smoking can raise blood pressure even more than nicotine does on its own.

Smoking also damages the body in other ways. The chemicals absorbed from tobacco smoke affect the inner walls of your arteries, making them stiff and

WHEN YOU QUIT, YOU WIN

Many people continue to smoke because they think they can't undo the damage already done to their bodies. Or they know too many other smokers who have tried to stop and failed. These assumptions are wrong.

Your body has an incredible capacity to repair itself. Just 20 minutes after you quit smoking, your heart rate and blood pressure start to drop. After one or two days, the level of carbon monoxide in your blood drops to normal. Between two weeks and three months after quitting, your circulation will improve and your lungs will work better. Between one and 12 months after you quit, you won't cough as much or feel as short of breath. You'll also notice an improved sense of smell, and food will taste better to you. And most important, quitting cigarettes can add 10 years to your life!

Few smokers can quit smoking on the first try. But stopping smoking is like learning anything else new. It often takes several attempts, and one bad experience shouldn't keep you from trying again. In fact, you can learn from previous attempts, increasing your chances for being successful in the future.

You can also enhance your chances for success by getting help from your health care team or by using a program that specializes in helping smokers stop. Combining counseling and medications is the most effective way to quit smoking. Many safe medications can help you quit.

It's true that many people gain weight after stopping smoking. But the negative consequences of the added weight are more than offset by the positive health benefits of stopping smoking.

unable to expand. Over time, this leaves them more prone to the buildup of fatty deposits (plaques) that permanently narrow the arteries. Tobacco also triggers the release of hormones that cause the body to retain fluid. Both factors can lead to higher blood pressure.

Exposure to secondhand smoke is also a serious health hazard. It can cause lung cancer in nonsmokers and has been linked to heart disease in adults and sudden infant death syndrome, asthma attacks and ear infections in children. There is no safe level of exposure to secondhand smoke.

Each year in the United States, 34,000 nonsmokers die of heart disease caused by secondhand smoke. If you have other risk factors for heart disease, you must avoid secondhand smoke. Even without other risk factors, exposure to second-hand smoke is hazardous.

HOW STOPPING SMOKING HELPS YOUR BLOOD PRESSURE

Not smoking may only slightly reduce your usual blood pressure. But it's still important to stop. Here's why.

First, smoking can interfere with some blood pressure medications, keeping them from working as well as they should. Smoking sometimes prevents them from working at all. Second, having high blood pressure puts you at a higher risk of heart attack, heart failure and stroke because of the damage it can cause to your circulatory and neurological systems. Smoking

also damages arteries, adding to the cardiovascular risk high blood pressure poses to the heart. Put simply, when you combine high blood pressure with smoking, your odds of heart disease are much greater.

Breaking tobacco's grip

Some people can simply stop and never smoke again. Most people require several tries. But you can stop; most people who have ever smoked have successfully quit. And as you try, make sure to work with your health care team to stay in control of your blood pressure.

Becoming tobacco-free is a result of planning and commitment, not luck. The two strategies that have been shown to be most effective are behavioral counseling by a counselor or tobacco treatment specialist, and medication.

All smokers are not alike. Work with your health care team to develop a treatment plan that combines various strategies for:
- Coping with the symptoms of nicotine withdrawal.
- Improving overall physical and emotional health.
- Gaining social support and guidance, when necessary.
- Resisting the urge to smoke.

Don't expect to find and use a ready-made treatment plan. No single plan works for everybody — there's no "right way" to stop smoking. Build a stop plan that suits your needs. Using more than one strategy increases your chances of success. Eating better, exercising, getting enough sleep and reducing stress are all helpful strategies.

Almost everyone experiences some symptoms of nicotine withdrawal when stopping smoking. For most smokers, the symptoms last for a few weeks, becoming less intense and less frequent over time. Common symptoms include irritability, anxiety, nervousness and loss of focus. Using one or more kinds of medication may help ease these symptoms.

Many weeks after your stop date, you may still have the desire to light up, particularly in familiar smoking situations such as after a meal. These urges and cravings are generally brief, but can be very strong and hard to resist.

Certain strategies in your treatment plan may be to change behaviors or avoid situations that cause you to smoke. You may also identify alternative activities or distractions that help you resist the urges and cravings.

Most people who quit smoking relapse within the first three months. Often, people relapse because they get an overwhelming urge to smoke and haven't developed a "fire escape" plan.

The following guidelines can increase your chances of success:

Do your homework

Read about the dangers of tobacco products and talk to people who have stopped or are trying to stop smoking. Think about your smoking behaviors and plan for ways to prevent or avoid them. Consider why you want to give up cigarettes. This preparation will help you when the day finally comes to stop smoking.

Set a stop day

Although setting a firm date to stop smoking is best, you can choose to cut back gradually as long as you have a stop date set in the foreseeable future. Carefully select a day when you throw your cigarettes away and no longer light up. It's unlikely that you'll have a time when you're totally stress-free, so don't let this get in the way of setting and sticking to your stop date.

Consider medication and counseling

Medications are available that can lessen nicotine withdrawal symptoms and increase your comfort and sense of control as you work toward becoming tobacco-free. They include bupropion and varenicline. Medications can't do all the work, but they can provide you with a better chance of success.

Research suggests that medication paired with counseling from a trained health care professional is even more effective than medication on its own. Ask your health care team about counseling services. In addition, many states and health organizations have telephone quit lines that provide advice and counseling.

Some provide free nicotine patches or nicotine gum. Online programs from the American Lung Association and the American Cancer Society can also help.

Tell others about your decision to stop

The support of family, friends and coworkers can help you reach your goal sooner. But many smokers choose to keep their plans a secret. That's because they don't want to look like a failure if they return to smoking. Keep in mind that it's better to be open and honest with yourself and those who support you.

Remember, it can take many tries before you may stop smoking for good. So there's no reason to feel like a failure just because your effort doesn't work out this time. Enlisting the support of at least one person can help you through a lapse.

Avoid smoking situations

Stay away from situations in which you used to smoke. Leave the table right after a meal if this was a time when you used to light up and go for a walk instead. If you always smoked while you talked on the phone with friends, avoid long phone conversations or change the location where you talk. If you had a favorite smoking chair, don't sit in it anymore.

For many people, avoiding alcohol in the first weeks of an attempt to quit smoking is an important strategy. And avoid secondhand smoke — it can be a powerful trigger to smoke.

To some degree, you'll be able to tell when you're about to feel the urge to smoke. Before it hits, start doing something that makes smoking inconvenient, such as making the bed, clearing the dinner table or washing the dishes. Smoking behavior is deeply ingrained and automatic — so you need to anticipate your reflex response to this urge and plan alternatives.

Change your routine

Try to reduce the number of routine activities or situations that you identify with smoking before your stop day. That will make it easier to stop completely. For example, stop smoking inside your car or your house. This will help you become more comfortable being in those places without smoking.

You can also reduce the number of cigarettes you smoke before your stop day, but remember that your goal is to stop completely.

Get regular physical activity.

Many studies have shown that starting a regular exercise program helps people to quit smoking.

Take one day at a time

On your stop day, stop completely and on each day following, focus on staying tobacco-free. Don't worry about tomorrow, next week or the rest of your life.

Just take it one day at a time, one urge at a time.

Time each urge

Check your watch when an urge to smoke hits. Most are short. Once you realize this, it may be easier to resist. Remind yourself, "I can make it another few minutes, and then the urge will pass."

Use medications along with other strategies to stop smoking

Remember that medications are just one part of your overall plan.

ALCOHOL AND BLOOD PRESSURE

There's a clear link between how much alcohol you drink and its effect on your

---

WHAT ABOUT CAFFEINE?

Caffeine is a mild stimulant found in coffee, tea, soft drinks and chocolate. It can fight fatigue, improve concentration and lighten mood. But too much caffeine can cause jitters, trembling hands and even possibly increase blood pressure.

The amount of caffeine in about two cups of coffee has been shown to raise blood pressure for a few hours. If you don't consume coffee regularly, in particular, or you if consume more than you usually do, you may experience a temporary spike in blood pressure. Exactly what causes it is unknown.

However, regularly drinking caffeinated beverages doesn't mean you're destined to develop high blood pressure. Some people who regularly drink caffeinated beverages have a higher average blood pressure than those who drink none. Others who regularly drink caffeinated beverages develop a tolerance to caffeine. As a result, caffeine doesn't have a long-term effect on their blood pressure.

As a general precaution, many health care professionals advise people with high blood pressure to limit daily caffeine intake to no more than 300 mg a day to prevent any effects. That's the amount in about three 8-oz. cups of coffee or six 8-oz. cups of black tea. You may even want to cut back more, to 200 mg of caffeine a day, or about two cups of coffee or four cups of black tea.

In addition, it's good practice to avoid caffeine right before activities that naturally increase your blood pressure, such as exercise or hard physical labor. Limiting caffeine is generally recommended.

blood pressure. While small amounts of alcohol don't seem to increase blood pressure, drinking too much can increase blood pressure and interfere with how well blood pressure-lowering medication works.

Exactly how excess alcohol increases blood pressure is unknown. One theory is that alcohol consumption triggers the late release of epinephrine (adrenaline) and other hormones that constrict your blood vessels or cause your kidneys to retain more sodium and water, generally after the effect of the alcohol wears off. This, in turn, raises your blood pressure.

Excessive drinking is also associated with poor nutrition, which can deplete your levels of the minerals that help control blood pressure.

It's not only the amount of alcohol you consume but also when you consume it that matters. A recent study suggests that people who drink alcohol at other times than with meals will have a much higher risk of high blood pressure, no matter how much they drink.

Regardless of how excess alcohol affects blood pressure, it's clear that reducing alcohol consumption lowers blood pressure. Heavy drinkers who cut back to moderate levels can lower systolic blood pressure by about 7 to 12 mm Hg and diastolic pressure by about 3 mm Hg. If you drink alcohol, the best advice is to do so only in moderation. For women, this is no more than one drink a day. For most men, moderate drinking is up to two drinks a day. One drink is equal to one 12-ounce bottle of beer, one 5-ounce glass

KEY POINTS

- If you have high blood pressure and you smoke tobacco products, your risk of death from a heart attack, heart failure or stroke is much higher than if you don't smoke.
- It takes planning and commitment to stop smoking. Develop your own stop plan with coping skills, social support and strategies to deal with the symptoms of nicotine withdrawal.
- For many people, moderate alcohol use doesn't seem to affect blood pressure, but excessive alcohol use can have serious consequences for your cardiovascular system.
- Alcohol use may interfere with some high blood pressure medications or increase their side effects.
- Caffeine can cause a temporary but sharp rise in blood pressure, particularly among people who don't regularly consume caffeine. If you have high blood pressure, you may want to limit daily caffeine intake.

of wine or one 1.5-ounce shot glass of 80-proof liquor.

Though some evidence suggests that moderate drinking may offer benefits, there's no reason to start drinking alcohol now if you don't drink already.

Alcohol and medications

If you take blood pressure medication, pay attention to when you consume alcohol. Alcohol can interfere with the effectiveness of some high blood pressure medications and increase their side effects. If you mix alcohol with a beta blocker, which relaxes your blood vessels and slows your heart rate, you may feel lightheaded or faint — especially if you're overheated or if you stand up suddenly.

You can experience the same symptoms if you drink alcohol close to the time you take an angiotensin-converting enzyme (ACE) inhibitor or certain calcium channel blockers. If you feel dizzy or faint, sit until the feeling passes. Drinking water also may help. In general, avoid drinking alcohol if you're taking any medication that causes drowsiness. Read the medication label before you consume alcohol.

And listen to your body. If you feel lightheaded or depressed after a drink or two, talk to your health care team.

Taking the right medication

8

Although lifestyle changes are the first choice for lowering blood pressure, medication is often needed.

For example, maybe you have stage 1 hypertension — a systolic pressure (the top number in your blood pressure reading) between 130 and 139 millimeters of mercury (mm Hg) and a diastolic pressure (the bottom number in your blood pressure reading) between 80 and 89 mm Hg. You've tried making lifestyle changes, but after a few months, you haven't been able to lower your blood pressure to a healthy level.

At the same time, maybe your risk of a heart attack or stroke in the next 10 years is high. This is something your health care team can calculate. In this situation, you'd likely need medication.

If you have stage 2 hypertension — a systolic pressure of 140 mm Hg or greater or a diastolic pressure of 90 mm Hg or greater — you may need medication right away, even with lifestyle changes. That's because medication can lower blood pressure further, and more quickly, than lifestyle changes can. You may also need medication if you have other conditions in addition to high blood pressure.

In this chapter, you'll learn about medications used to lower blood pressure.

Blood pressure medications (antihypertensives) are a major success story in modern medicine. They're quite effective, and most people aren't bothered by their side effects. These drugs can allow you to live well with controlled blood pressure. They can also reduce risks related to other health conditions.

MANY OPTIONS

There are several classes of blood pressure medication, and each class affects blood pressure in a different way.

The major classes of medication used to control high blood pressure include:
- Diuretics
- Beta blockers
- Angiotensin-converting enzyme (ACE) inhibitors
- Angiotensin II receptor blockers (ARBs)
- Renin inhibitors
- Calcium channel blockers (calcium antagonists)
- Alpha blockers
- Alpha-beta blockers
- Central-acting agents
- Vasodilators
- Aldosterone antagonists

How these medications are prescribed is based on several factors, starting with your blood pressure level and risk of a heart attack or stroke. Many other factors also play a role in medication choice.

Finding the right medication or combination of medications may take time. Your age, ethnicity and overall health, other medications you are taking, how often you take the drugs, how you feel when you take them, and the total cost of the medication are all factors to consider.

If you're prescribed one drug but it doesn't lower your blood pressure to a safe level, your health care team may substitute a drug from a different class of medications or add another medication to your prescription. Together, two or more low-dose drugs may lower your blood pressure as well as or better than one drug alone can at full dose. Using lower

DIURETICS AND YOUR KIDNEYS

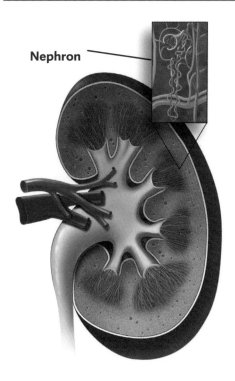

Nephron

Tiny bundles of intertwining blood vessels and tubules called nephrons are the filtering units of the kidneys. Each kidney is packed with about 1 million of them. Different types of diuretics act on different parts of the nephron.

doses of medications together may also cause fewer side effects.

Sometimes it's possible to treat two or more conditions with one medication, so talk with your health care team about any other conditions you have. What's most important is that you're working with your health care team to develop a treatment plan that's tolerable, cost-effective and personalized.

With this background in mind, here's a general look at how blood pressure medications are prescribed.

Medications prescribed first

The first medications usually prescribed to treat high blood pressure are thiazide diuretics, ACE inhibitors, angiotensin II receptor blockers and calcium channel blockers. Here's more on each type.

Thiazide diuretics

Diuretics were first introduced in the 1950s and are still commonly used to lower blood pressure. Known as water pills, diuretics reduce the volume of fluid in the body. They tell the kidneys to excrete more sodium in the urine than they usually do. The sodium takes with it water from the blood so that there's a smaller volume of blood pushing through the arteries. This means less pressure on the artery walls. Diuretics also cause the blood vessels to open (dilate), which reduces blood pressure. Diuretics are often the first medication prescribed for

people with stage 1 hypertension. They're highly effective in Black people and in older adults, who more often are sodium sensitive. Diuretics are also commonly used along with other medications.

Compared to other high blood pressure drugs, diuretics have two major advantages. First, they're less expensive than other blood pressure drugs. Second, they've repeatedly proved their effectiveness over the years. For example, in the Antihypertensive and Lipid-Lowering Treatment to Prevent Heart Attack Trial (ALLHAT), researchers found that among about 33,000 people age 55 and older, diuretics were more effective than ACE inhibitors or calcium channel blockers in controlling high blood pressure and preventing heart disease. A later study reaffirmed these conclusions.

If you take a diuretic, it's important to also limit sodium and get enough potassium in your diet. These steps will help the drug work more effectively and with fewer side effects.

There are three types of diuretics, but only thiazide diuretics are prescribed as a first-line medication to treat high blood pressure. You'll learn when the other two types are prescribed later in this chapter.

In addition to controlling high blood pressure, thiazide diuretics provide other potential benefits. They've been shown to reduce the risk of stroke, heart attack and heart failure. They also reduce the amount of calcium in the urine, so kidney stones are less likely to form. With less calcium in your urine, more calcium stays in your blood, helping to reduce your risk of osteoporosis and hip fracture.

Types of thiazide diuretics

Thiazide and thiazide-like diuretics include:
- Chlorothiazide (Diuril)
- Chlorthalidone (Thalitone)
- Hydrochlorothiazide (Microzide)
- Indapamide
- Metolazone

Side effects and cautions

The most common side effect of diuretics is needing to urinate more. Thiazide diuretics can also cause low potassium levels, so they're often used with an ACE inhibitor or an angiotensin II receptor blocker, which you'll learn about next; or a potassium-sparing diuretic, which you'll learn about later in this chapter.

In rare cases, your magnesium level may need to be corrected before your potassium level is addressed. That's because changes in magnesium may worsen changes in potassium.

In older adults, diuretics may also cause dizziness upon standing. Although it's uncommon, these medications can also cause erectile dysfunction (impotence, or ED) in some men. In high doses, thiazides can slightly increase blood sugar and cholesterol levels. They also increase the level of uric acid in the blood. In rare cases, this can lead to a joint disorder called gout.

Thiazides can also cause a rare condition known as hyponatremia. This condition involves low levels of sodium in the blood. It often occurs in older adults who take thiazide diuretics and drink too much water. Hyponatremia causes headaches and confusion and can lead to a coma.

You may need your sodium, potassium and creatinine levels checked a couple of weeks after you start taking a diuretic.

ACE inhibitors

Angiotensin-converting enzyme (ACE) inhibitors help reduce blood pressure by preventing the enzyme from producing angiotensin II. This substance causes the blood vessels to contract and stimulates release of the hormone aldosterone (see an illustration of the process on page 13).

Limiting the action of the angiotensin-converting enzyme also allows another substance called bradykinin — which keeps blood vessels open (dilated) — to remain in the bloodstream, reducing blood pressure.

ACE inhibitors are a common choice for treating high blood pressure because they're effective and produce few side effects. Among Black people, ACE inhibitors are most effective when they're combined with a diuretic.

In addition to lowering blood pressure, ACE inhibitors help prevent and treat cardiovascular disease, including coronary artery disease, left ventricular hypertrophy, heart failure and stroke.

The drugs also delay progression of kidney disease and may protect against diabetes.

Types of ACE inhibitors

ACE inhibitors include:
- Benazepril (Lotensin)
- Captopril
- Enalapril (Vasotec, Epaned)
- Fosinopril
- Lisinopril (Zestril, Qbrelis)
- Moexipril
- Perindopril
- Quinapril (Accupril)
- Ramipril (Altace)
- Trandolapril

Side effects and cautions

ACE inhibitors generally cause few side effects. However, it can cause a dry cough. This occurs more often in women than it does in men. In some people, the cough sticks around long enough and is annoying enough to warrant switching to another medication. ACE inhibitors may also cause a rise in potassium, which can be dangerous if gets too high. This is mainly a concern for people who have chronic kidney disease or diabetes.

Other possible side effects may include rash, altered sense of taste and reduced appetite. For some people and in some situations, ACE inhibitor use requires special consideration and attention. In addition, ACE inhibitors aren't recommended for those who are pregnant or plan to become pregnant because the drugs can cause birth defects.

Rarely — but more commonly in Black people and in people who smoke — this medication may cause small areas of tissue swelling (angioedema). Swelling in the throat can be life-threatening.

Angiotensin II receptor blockers

Angiotensin II receptor blockers (ARBs) block the action of the chemical angiotensin II, as compared to ACE inhibitors, which keep angiotensin II from forming. Angiotensin II receptor blockers also differ from ACE inhibitors in that they don't affect the levels of bradykinin, which keeps blood vessels open (dilated).

Studies suggest that ARBs work about as well as ACE inhibitors in treating high blood pressure and heart failure. ARBs can be used to treat heart disease, including coronary artery disease and stroke. They rarely cause a dry cough.

Types of angiotensin II receptor blockers

Angiotensin II receptor blockers include:
- Azilsartan (Edarbi)
- Candesartan (Atacand)
- Irbesartan (Avapro)
- Losartan (Cozaar)
- Olmesartan (Benicar)
- Telmisartan (Micardis)
- Valsartan (Diovan)

Side effects and cautions

Side effects are uncommon, but in some people, ARBs can cause dizziness, nasal congestion, diarrhea, indigestion and insomnia. In rare cases, ARBs may cause certain tissues in the body to swell. Those who are pregnant or may become pregnant shouldn't take these drugs. Olmesartan has also been reported to cause gastrointestinal issues that resolve with stopping the medication.

Calcium channel blockers

Also called calcium antagonists, calcium channel blockers affect the muscle cells in the walls of the arteries. These muscle cells contain tiny passages in their membranes called calcium channels. When calcium carried in the bloodstream flows into them, the muscle cells contract and the arteries narrow. Calcium channel blockers keep calcium from getting into the muscle cells by blocking the channels.

Calcium channel blockers don't affect the levels of calcium used by your body to build bone and maintain your musculoskeletal system. They work well and are generally well tolerated. They may work better for Black people than drugs such as beta blockers, ACE inhibitors and angiotensin II receptor blockers.

Some calcium channel blockers offer the added benefit of slowing heart rate, potentially reducing blood pressure, relieving a type of chest pain called angina and controlling irregular heartbeat. Calcium channel blockers have also been shown to help prevent migraines and Raynaud's disease, which affects blood circulation in your hands and feet.

These drugs are one of the four classes of drugs recommended first to treat high blood pressure. They're often preferred for Black people and older people with systolic hypertension.

Types of calcium channel blockers

Long-acting calcium channel blockers include:
- Amlodipine (Norvasc)
- Diltiazem (Cardizem, Tiazac, others)*
- Felodipine
- Isradipine
- Nicardipine

I'M AFRAID OF MEDICATION SIDE EFFECTS. WHAT CAN I DO?

Because a medication can cause side effects doesn't mean you'll experience them. Side effects are generally reported among only a small number of users. Talk to your health care team about any concerns you have. There are ways to test your reaction to a drug, for example, by starting at a low dose and gradually raising the dose. Also, many side effects tend to lessen after a short amount of use.

- Nifedipine (Procardia)
- Nisoldipine (Sular)
- Verapamil (Calan SR, Verelan)*

*These drugs also slow heart rate, can treat certain heart arrhythmias and angina, and prevent second heart attacks and migraines.

Side effects and cautions

Possible side effects include constipation, headache, fast heartbeat, rash, swollen feet and lower legs, fatigue, flushing and nausea. It's important to not consume grapefruit, grapefruit juice, sour oranges or pomelos if you're taking felodipine, nifedipine, nisoldipine or verapamil. A substance in the juice of these fruits seems to impair how well these medications are broken down (metabolized), allowing them to build up in the body and become toxic.

If you need more than one drug

If the medication you're taking doesn't lower your blood pressure enough, you're not alone. Research shows that most people with high blood pressure need two or more medications to get their blood pressure to a healthy level.

If your blood pressure medication isn't working, your health care team may first increase the dosage if you aren't experiencing any significant side effects. Or you may try a completely different drug. Another option is to add a second drug to the one you're already taking — an

approach known as combination drug therapy. Your health care team will likely add a medication from those you've already learned about. For example, if you're taking a thiazide diuretic and need a second medication to control your blood pressure, you may take an ACE inhibitor or an ARB.

If your blood pressure still isn't controlled with two medications, you may add a calcium channel blocker.

When three medications aren't enough

It's only in rare cases that medications fail to lower high blood pressure to the targeted goal. Often, it just takes time and trials with different drugs and doses to find the combination that works best.

But what if you've been following your health care team's advice, watching your weight, getting exercise and taking your medication, but still aren't able to lower your blood pressure?

Many times, the first step is to try a different type of drug or a different combination of drugs in a single medication. A combination of drugs in a single formulation reduces the number of pills needed a day and can help you stick with your medication routine. Some medications simply work better for some people than for others.

The next step may be to add another medication to the one you're already taking, perhaps a third or even a fourth drug. Drugs working together can have a more powerful effect on blood pressure than they do when taken separately.

Common issues include inadequate diuretic therapy or the need for a more powerful diuretic, such as a loop diuretic. Here's more on the medications that may be prescribed at this point.

Loop diuretics and potassium-sparing diuretics

Thiazide diuretics are one of the medications often prescribed first for high blood pressure. If you need additional medication to lower blood pressure, you may take two other types of diuretics: loop diuretics and potassium-sparing diuretics.

Types of loop diuretics and potassium-sparing diuretics

Loop diuretics include:
- Bumetanide (Bumex)
- Ethacrynic acid (Edecrin)
- Furosemide (Lasix)
- Torsemide (Soaanz)

Potassium-sparing diuretics include:
- Amiloride (Midamor)
- Eplerenone (Inspra)
- Spironolactone (Aldactone, CaroSpir)
- Triamterene (Dyrenium)

Side effects and cautions

Loop diuretics remove more sodium from the kidneys than thiazide diuretics. They may also remove more calcium, although

proper monitoring can prevent complications. Your health care team may recommend a loop diuretic if thiazides aren't effective, particularly if you have chronic kidney disease or other conditions that cause your body to retain fluid.

In addition to removing sodium from the blood, thiazide and loop diuretics remove potassium. Potassium-sparing diuretics help the body retain needed potassium, as their name suggests.

Potassium-sparing diuretics aren't as powerful as other diuretics, so they're often used alongside them. When taken with other medications, the potassium-sparing diuretic spironolactone also helps people with heart failure live longer and is particularly effective with resistant high blood pressure. Eplerenone is an improved version of spironolactone that appears to have fewer side effects.

As with thiazide diuretics, the most common side effect of potassium-sparing and loop diuretics is increased urination. Loop diuretics can also cause low potassium levels, so they're often used with a potassium-sparing diuretic, ACE inhibitor or ARB. In rare cases, your magnesium level may need to be corrected before your potassium level is addressed.

Potassium-sparing diuretics may raise your potassium level too much. Blood tests can detect this. If your kidney function is impaired, you shouldn't take a potassium-sparing diuretic.

Your health care team may want to check your sodium, potassium and creatinine levels a few weeks after you start taking a diuretic.

Beta blockers

Beta blockers lower blood pressure by blocking many of the effects of the hormone epinephrine, also known as adrenaline. This action makes your heart beat more slowly and less forcefully, helping to lower your blood pressure.

Beta blockers also slowly lower the kidneys' release of the enzyme renin. As you learned earlier, renin is involved in the production of a substance called angiotensin II, which narrows the blood vessels and increases blood pressure. (For a reminder of how this works, see page 120.)

Like diuretics, beta blockers have been used for many years and they lower blood pressure in most people who take them.

Beta blockers alone may not be the first choice for cases of uncomplicated high blood pressure; they may be better used in combination with another drug option.

However, beta blockers are especially helpful if high blood pressure is accompanied by heart-related conditions such as chest pain (angina), irregular heart rhythm (arrhythmia), heart failure or previous heart attack. They help control these conditions and reduce your risk of a second heart attack.

Beta blockers are often used in older adults with heart disease. Black people don't respond as well as white people to most beta blockers as a single drug.

These drugs were first developed to treat coronary artery disease and were later approved to treat high blood pressure after studies found they could lower it. They may also be used to treat migraines, anxiety, hyperthyroidism and some tremors. These drugs are often chosen for people with high blood pressure who are or may become pregnant.

Types of beta blockers

Beta blockers can affect the heart (cardioselective) or both the heart and blood vessels (noncardioselective). Cardioselective drugs generally produce fewer side effects.

Cardioselective beta blockers include:
• Acebutolol
• Atenolol (Tenormin)
• Betaxolol
• Bisoprolol
• Nebivolol (Bystolic)
• Metoprolol (Lopressor, Toprol XL)

Noncardioselective types include:
• Nadolol (Corgard)
• Pindolol
• Propranolol (Inderal LA, InnoPran XL)
• Timolol

Drugs that combine an alpha blocker and a beta blocker are listed on page 129. If you have liver or kidney problems, your choice of beta blockers may be limited. Beta blockers are broken down in the liver, kidneys, or both.

If the kidneys aren't working properly, for example, a beta blocker that's usually removed by the kidneys may build to toxic levels.

Side effects and cautions

Although side effects may occur when taking beta blockers, many people who take beta blockers won't have any.

Two notable side effects of beta blockers are feeling tired and feeling less able to take part in strenuous physical activity. Other side effects may include cold hands, trouble sleeping, erectile dysfunction (impotence, or ED), loss of sex drive, a slight rise in triglycerides, slight weight gain and a small decrease in high-density lipoprotein (HDL, or "good") cholesterol.

If you're an active person or an athlete, beta blockers won't be your first choice of treatment because they can limit your ability to be fully active. They're also not recommended for people with asthma or a severe blockage in the conducting system of the heart.

Renin inhibitor

The renin inhibitor aliskiren (Tekturna) blocks an enzyme in the body that produces a substance (angiotensin II) that causes blood vessels to tighten. As a result, the blood vessels relax. This decreases the blood pressure. This medication affects this process at a much earlier stage than do other drugs.

Though side effects are uncommon, they include diarrhea and an allergic reaction that causes face swelling and trouble breathing. One important note: Don't use aliskiren if you are pregnant or if you may become pregnant.

Alpha blockers

Alpha blockers reduce the effect of the hormone norepinephrine (noradrenaline), which stimulates muscles in the walls of smaller arteries. As a result, the walls don't narrow as much as they might usually. For older people with prostate problems, alpha blockers also improve urine flow and reduce the number of

ALPHA-BETA BLOCKERS

Certain drugs combine the effects of an alpha blocker and a beta blocker. Alpha-beta blockers such as carvedilol (Coreg, Coreg CR) and labetalol lower blood pressure by reducing nerve impulses like alpha blockers and slowing the heartbeat like beta blockers. The same precautions are necessary for these drugs as for beta blockers and alpha blockers. Possible side effects include fatigue, dizziness, slow heartbeat and increased blood sugar.

awakenings at night to go to the bathroom. Alpha blockers have been used to treat hypertension for more than two decades. They used to be prescribed on their own, but now are used with other high blood pressure drugs. Alpha blockers aren't recommended as one of the first drugs to treat high blood pressure.

Types of alpha blockers

Alpha blockers are available in both short-acting and long-acting forms. Alpha blockers include:
- Doxazosin (Cardura, Cardura XL), a long-acting drug
- Terazosin, a long-acting drug

COMBINING DRUGS IN ONE PILL

If you're taking more than one drug and have established a medication regimen that's working well for you, you may consider taking tablets that combine medications for convenience. They may cost more than buying each medication separately but can be more convenient. Taking one pill rather than several can make it easier to take your medications regularly and help you achieve better blood pressure control.

A combination pill can also help you manage more than one condition at the same time. One example is the combination drug Caduet, which combines amlodipine, a calcium channel blocker, with atorvastatin, a statin used to treat high cholesterol. Since high blood pressure and high cholesterol are often present at the same time, both conditions can be treated conveniently with a single medication.

Another benefit of combination drugs is that you may be using them at lower doses. For example, certain blood pressure medications, such as thiazide diuretics and statins, increase the risk of new-onset diabetes when used at higher doses or for long duration. The use of these drugs at lower doses in combination with another medication can offset this risk, especially if potassium is kept at a healthy level.

Following are examples of these combination drugs:

ACE inhibitor and diuretic
- Benazepril and hydrochlorothiazide (Lotensin HCT).
- Enalapril and hydrochlorothiazide (Vaseretic).
- Lisinopril and hydrochlorothiazide (Zestoretic).

- Prazosin (Minipress), a short-acting drug

Side effects and cautions

Alpha blockers generally cause few side effects and should be taken just before bedtime.

However, when you first begin taking them or if you're older, they may cause you to feel dizzy or faint when you stand up. That's because alpha blockers slow the time it takes the body to respond to natural changes in blood pressure when you move from a sitting or lying position to a standing position. Other possible side

ARB and diuretic
- Losartan and hydrochlorothiazide (Hyzaar).
- Valsartan and hydrochlorothiazide (Diovan HCT).

Beta blocker and diuretic
- Atenolol and chlorthalidone (Tenoretic).
- Bisoprolol and hydrochlorothiazide (Ziac).
- Metoprolol and hydrochlorothiazide (Lopressor HCT).

Two diuretics
- Amiloride and hydrochlorothiazide.
- Spironolactone and hydrochlorothiazide (Aldactazide).
- Triamterene and hydrochlorothiazide (Maxzide).

Calcium channel blocker and ACE inhibitor
- Amlodipine and benazepril (Lotrel).
- Verapamil and trandolapril.

ARB and calcium channel blocker
- Valsartan and amlodipine (Exforge).

In some cases, combinations of three medications are used to treat hypertension.

effects include headache, pounding heartbeat and weakness.

Central-acting agents

Unlike other blood pressure drugs that work mostly on the heart and blood vessels, these drugs work on the nervous system. Central-acting agents prevent centers in the brain from signaling the nerves to speed up heart rate and narrow blood vessels. As a result, the heart doesn't pump as hard, which helps blood flow more easily through the arteries.

Also called central adrenergic inhibitors, central-acting agents aren't used often because they can produce strong side effects. However, they're still sometimes prescribed. They may be recommended for individuals who have hot flashes, attention-deficit/hyperactivity disorder (ADHD) and Tourette syndrome, and for people who are going through drug withdrawal, such as from opioid pain medications.

One central-acting agent, clonidine, is available as a skin patch, which is helpful if you have trouble taking pills. Another agent, methyldopa, is often recommended for pregnant people with high blood pressure.

Types of central-acting agents

Central-acting agents include:
- Clonidine (Catapres-TTS, Kapvay)
- Guanfacine (Intuniv)
- Methyldopa

Side effects and cautions

Central-acting agents can cause extreme fatigue, drowsiness and dizziness. They can also cause erectile dysfunction (impotence, or ED), dry mouth, a slow heart rate, constipation, fever and headache. Stopping the use of these drugs can cause blood pressure to rise quickly to dangerously high levels.

If you're bothered by side effects, don't stop taking the medication on your own. Ask your health care team about the best way to quit using it gradually.

HOW CAN I REDUCE MY MEDICATION COSTS?

Following a healthy lifestyle program can reduce the number of medications or the dosage required to reach and maintain your blood pressure goals. Often, after medications have helped control your blood pressure for some months, it may be possible to slowly taper down the dosage — but do this only under your health care team's guidance. Also, ask about generic equivalent medications. It may also be possible to receive assistance with cost from the manufacturer. For more on cost savings, see Chapter 10.

Direct vasodilators

These potent medications are used mostly to treat high blood pressure that doesn't respond well to other drugs. They work on the muscles in the walls of the arteries and veins. They keep these muscles from tightening and the walls from narrowing.

Types of direct vasodilators

Direct vasodilators prescribed to work directly on the vessel walls are hydralazine and minoxidil.

Side effects and cautions

Among their possible side effects, the most common are a fast heartbeat and fluid retention — neither of which is desirable if you have high blood pressure. That's why they're typically prescribed with a beta blocker and diuretic. This helps make these symptoms less likely.

Other side effects may include nausea, vomiting, headache, joint pain and chest pain. Minoxidil also may result in excessive hair growth. Hydralazine can increase the risk of lupus, an autoimmune disorder that affects connective tissues.

HOW THE BODY PROCESSES DRUGS CAN MAKE A DIFFERENCE

People are either rapid, normal or slow metabolizers. If you're a slow metabolizer, a drug may build up in the body, possibly making you more prone to side effects because it sticks around in the body longer. If you're a fast metabolizer, a drug may not have much of an effect on blood pressure because the body gets rid of it too quickly.

Genotype testing helps show how quickly you metabolize certain drugs based on the enzyme systems used to process them. This testing isn't done right away for every medication. Instead, this kind of testing is mostly done in a troubleshooting phase after a drug has been started, if it isn't working in the way it's supposed to. In some cases, though, certain drugs can have lethal consequences if they're metabolized too slowly — and in those cases, genotype testing is done before someone starts taking a drug.

The point of all this, with regard to blood pressure medication, is that if it isn't working well, your health care team may suggest genotype testing to see if you're metabolizing it too quickly. Or you may have this kind of testing to see if another drug you're taking for a different condition is affecting how the body metabolizes the blood pressure medication you're taking, making it less effective.

HELP YOUR HEALTH CARE TEAM HELP YOU

For most people, high blood pressure can be controlled with three medications. However, for a small number of people, this isn't the case.

If you're taking three medications and your blood pressure still isn't under control, talk with your health care team. Be honest about the challenges you're facing. Are you struggling to remember to take your medications? Are you having trouble affording your medications? Are you experiencing side effects? Do you have sleep apnea or another condition that's keeping your blood pressure high? Is your diet — or are other medications you're taking — keeping your blood pressure drugs from working as they should? Your health care team can help you work through these and other issues.

If your blood pressure hasn't responded to drug therapy, ask yourself:

- *Have I been taking my medication exactly as prescribed?* Take your medication exactly as prescribed, or it may not work. If you think the pills cost too much, if the regimen is too hard to follow or if the side effects of the medication are too unpleasant to live with, talk to your health care team. Other drugs may be a better match.

One note about once-a-day medications: They may not control blood pressure for a full 24 hours. This can be detected through home blood pressure monitoring. If this is the case for you, you'll need to take some of your medication at bedtime rather than taking all of it in the morning.

- *Am I telling my health care team about all the drugs and herbs I take?* Many medications and supplements, including over-the-counter products, may cause problems with blood pressure medication.
- *Am I drinking too much alcohol?* Alcohol can keep blood pressure high, especially if you consume a large amount within a short time. Your medication may not be able to overcome the effects of alcohol and alcohol may interfere with the action of the drug. Keep your alcohol use moderate. In general, that's no more than two drinks a day for most men and no more than one drink a day for women. For more information, see Chapter 7.
- *Have I seriously tried to stop smoking?* Like alcohol, tobacco products can keep blood pressure persistently high if you use them frequently. Quitting smoking can not only lower your blood pressure but can also reduce your risk of other types of heart disease. Learn more about the effects of tobacco and ways to quit in Chapter 7.
- *Have I gained weight?* Generally, losing weight lowers blood pressure. Weight gain — as few as 10 pounds — can increase it and make it harder to control.
- *Have I been sleeping well?* Sleep apnea can raise blood pressure (see page 146). The disorder occurs most frequently in older adults. Relieving sleep apnea can lower blood pressure.

If you and your health care team have exhausted these possibilities, you still

- Medication may be needed if lifestyle changes aren't effective, you have stage 2 high blood pressure or you have another medical condition that could benefit from drug use.
- While many people can control their blood pressure with just one drug, others need a combination of two or three drugs.
- Because of their proven success, diuretics, ACE inhibitors, ARBs or calcium channel blockers are often prescribed for uncomplicated high blood pressure. Beta blockers are being used less now than before as a single drug for high blood pressure, but more for certain conditions that may accompany the disorder.
- Finding the right drug or combination of drugs to control your blood pressure is a process that requires time and patience.

Other options include adding a fourth drug to your daily regimen or taking more of your current medication. Aldosterone blockers, in particular, can play an important role in cases of high blood pressure that's not responding to other drugs. The danger in increasing dosages is an increased risk of side effects from the medication. If you aren't already seeing a high blood pressure specialist, ask your health care team for a referral. See the Additional Resources section of this book for more information on finding high blood pressure specialists in your area.

THE RIGHT MEDICATION IS OUT THERE

Finding the right blood pressure drug or combination of medications is often a trial-and-error process. But almost everyone who takes blood pressure medication is able to come up with a drug regimen that allows them to reach their target goal. These drugs will allow you to feel good and be fully active. And they will produce few, if any, side effects.

have options. To start, you may need to step up the positive changes to your lifestyle. If you can walk another block, lose one more pound or improve your diet, your treatment may work better.

Reconsider the reversible causes of high blood pressure, including medications for other conditions, supplements or foods, sleep apnea or other conditions.

Special concerns and conditions

High blood pressure requires special care and consideration for certain people and in specific situations. This chapter focuses on factors unique to specific groups of people, as well as high blood pressure accompanied by other conditions. The course of treatment may vary in these situations.

Not too long ago, most studies on high blood pressure primarily examined its effect on men. Yet, nearly half of all Americans diagnosed with high blood pressure are women.

It's apparent that women often develop the disease for different reasons and at different times in their lives than do men. Women may have a different pattern of signs and symptoms and may respond differently to medication. More studies are focusing on issues that specifically affect women.

Oral contraceptives

Oral contraceptives — the pill — are a common form of birth control. The pill doesn't cause high blood pressure in most people who take it. But in some people, it can cause blood pressure to increase, especially for those who are over age 35, overweight or smokers.

If you develop high blood pressure while on the pill or have high blood pressure before you start taking it, consider a different form of birth control. If an alternative type of birth control isn't possible and you still want to take the pill, you'll need to have your blood pressure checked regularly and take steps to lower your blood pressure through lifestyle changes and possibly with the help of medication. When you stop taking the pill, it may take up to three months for your blood pressure to return to the level it was before you started taking the pill.

Birth control pills aren't recommended if you're over 35 and smoke, because their use increases the likelihood that you'll develop heart disease or have a stroke. Having high blood pressure in addition to these other factors can increase your risks even more.

A word of caution: A contraceptive that combines drospirenone and ethinyl estradiol (Yasmin, Yaz, others) contains a synthetic progestin that can cause you to retain potassium. This could lead to unusually high levels of potassium in your blood if you're also taking a potassium-sparing diuretic, angiotensin-converting enzyme (ACE) inhibitor, angiotensin II receptor blocker (ARB), aldosterone antagonist or other medication to manage your high blood pressure. Check with your health care team before combining birth control pills and high blood pressure medications.

Also, it's important to note that birth control pills containing drospirenone may be associated with a higher risk of blood clots, heart attack or stroke when compared to progestin-containing pills. Talk with your health care team about any concerns you have.

Pregnancy

It's quite possible for people with high blood pressure to have a healthy pregnancy and childbirth, but they should take precautions, starting with regularly scheduled checkups.

In a typical pregnancy, blood pressure gradually falls, reaching the lowest point around 22 to 24 weeks. Much of this decline happens early, within the first 6 to 8 weeks. Blood pressure then starts to rise during the third trimester and returns to prepregnancy levels at the time of delivery. Even in those with hypertension, blood pressure often lowers and then returns to its regular level during pregnancy. Blood pressure medication may be lowered or stopped altogether. In some people, blood pressure may not decline, while in others, it may increase.

If you have high blood pressure, you have a greater risk of complications during pregnancy, which can affect both you and your unborn child. As a result, your health care team will want to monitor your pregnancy and your blood pressure closely, especially during the last three months (the third trimester). This is when complications are most likely to occur.

Uncommon, but possible, complications for the mother include heart failure, stroke and other issues related to uncontrolled high blood pressure. Preeclampsia or eclampsia, potentially dangerous conditions that can occur during pregnancy, also may develop. (Read more about preeclampsia and eclampsia on pages 139-140.)

Possible complications for the baby include impaired growth, greater risk of the placenta separating from the uterine wall and greater risk of getting reduced levels of oxygen during labor. Some of these complications can require early delivery of the baby, either through induction or a C-section.

If you have high blood pressure before conceiving, talk with your health care team about the possible health risks of becoming pregnant. Your health care team may recommend changing your regimen, because some blood pressure medications shouldn't be taken during pregnancy.

Also, take measures to keep your blood pressure under control, such as getting regular physical activity, losing weight if you need to and taking your medication as prescribed.

Tell your health care team as soon as you become pregnant. One of the most important things you can do to have a healthy pregnancy is to get early and regular prenatal care. In addition to routine checkups, you may need regular blood and urine tests and frequent ultrasounds of the developing fetus.

If you see more than one health care professional for your care during your pregnancy, tell each person you see that you have high blood pressure. Because blood pressure usually decreases during the early and middle stages of pregnancy, someone who doesn't know your medical history may not realize you have high blood pressure.

If you need to take blood pressure medication during pregnancy, the central-acting drug methyldopa (Aldomet), labetalol (Trandate) or another type of beta blocker — or a calcium channel blocker — may be recommended.

At the same time, it's important to know which medications to avoid during pregnancy, which include angiotensin-converting enzyme (ACE) inhibitors, angiotensin II receptor blockers (ARBs) and renin inhibitors.

Gestational hypertension

A small number of people who don't have hypertension develop it during their pregnancies. It most often happens during the later stages of pregnancy, and the increase is usually slight. Once the pregnancy is complete, blood pressure returns to its prepregnancy level. If blood pressure doesn't bounce back to its usual level, that means high blood pressure was likely present before the pregnancy and was masked because blood pressure declined during pregnancy.

If you develop pregnancy-induced high blood pressure, especially if you remain within the stage 1 range, medication generally isn't necessary. But it will be important to follow a diet that emphasizes whole grains, fruits, vegetables and low-fat dairy products — foods that help control high blood pressure. Only if your blood pressure increases quite a bit — putting your health or your baby's health in jeopardy — is medication recommended.

Gestational hypertension is an early warning that you're at higher risk of hypertension and diseases related to it, such as heart disease or kidney disease, later in life.

Preeclampsia

Preeclampsia occurs in about 4% of pregnancies.

This condition is characterized by high blood pressure and signs of damage to another organ system, often the liver or kidneys. It typically develops after the 20th week of pregnancy.

Left untreated, preeclampsia can lead to serious, even deadly, complications. It can lead to kidney and liver damage, blood clotting issues and death. It's also been linked to premature birth and low birth weight in babies.

The exact cause of preeclampsia is unknown, but certain factors can increase risk. They include:
- Preexisting chronic high blood pressure
- First pregnancy
- Family history of preeclampsia
- Carrying multiple fetuses
- Diabetes
- Kidney problems before pregnancy
- Pregnancy at either end of the childbearing years — early teens or late 30s into 40s

Those who develop preeclampsia often have no symptoms at first. By the time they do appear, the condition may be advanced. Although swelling occurs in many pregnancies, obvious swelling in the face and hands and sudden weight gain of more than 2 pounds in a week due to fluid retention may be signs of this condition.

Other signs and symptoms include headache, vision problems and upper belly pain, usually under the ribs on the right side. If you experience any of these, talk to your health care team. Some of these signs and symptoms occur in typical pregnancies and don't mean that you have preeclampsia.

Your blood pressure and urine are checked routinely during your pregnancy. Your health care team also may perform blood tests to check your blood platelet count and to see how well your liver and kidneys are functioning. A low blood platelet level and increased liver enzyme values indicate a severe form of preeclampsia called HELLP (hemolysis, elevated liver enzymes and low platelet count) syndrome, which can become life-threatening.

If you have mild preeclampsia, your health care team will want to see you often to check your blood pressure and urine, do blood tests, and monitor your baby. You also may need to check your blood pressure at home. To prevent the condition from worsening, you may deliver your baby at 37 weeks instead of waiting until labor begins on its own.

Severe preeclampsia often requires a hospital stay so that your health and the health of your baby can be continuously monitored. You may be given medication to help control blood pressure and to prevent seizures. If your health or your baby's health may be at significant risk, early delivery may be necessary. Labor may be induced or a C-section may be performed.

After delivery, your blood pressure should return to its prepregnancy level within several days to several weeks. If your blood pressure is still at stage 2 when you leave the hospital with your baby, you may need to take blood pressure medication. You'll likely be able to taper off the medication after a few months.

The American Congress of Obstetricians and Gynecologists recommends low-dose aspirin for those who have a medical history of early-onset preeclampsia, preterm delivery at less than 34 weeks of gestation or preeclampsia in more than one previous pregnancy.

The U.S. Preventive Services Task Force recommends the use of low-dose aspirin, 81 mg daily, after 12 weeks' gestation for those at high risk of preeclampsia. Aspirin therapy is not recommended to prevent preeclampsia in those who are at a low risk of developing the condition.

Calcium supplements may also help prevent preeclampsia. Benefits are seen most in women with low calcium intake in their regular diet. The low risk and low cost of calcium supplements make them a good choice for those who are at high risk of preeclampsia. A dose of 1,000 milligrams (mg) a day is commonly recommended.

Eclampsia

Eclampsia is a life-threatening condition in which someone with preeclampsia has seizures. Signs and symptoms of eclampsia include:
- Pain in the upper right side of the belly.
- Severe headache and vision problems, including flashing lights in the field of vision.
- Convulsions.
- Altered mental status.
- Shortness of breath.
- Unconsciousness.

Eclampsia can damage the brain, liver or kidneys, and it can be fatal for both you and your unborn child. Emergency delivery of the baby is needed.

Menopause

Blood pressure generally increases after menopause, and so does the risk of high blood pressure. There has been some debate about whether these changes in blood pressure are truly due to menopause or are a consequence of age and weight gain.

Some health care experts think this increase suggests that shifting hormones related to menopause play a role. Other providers think an increase in body mass index (BMI) during menopause may be the more likely culprit.

It's a fact that before menopause, women have a slightly lower diastolic and systolic pressure than men of the same age. After menopause, systolic pressure in women increases by about 5 millimeters of mercury (mm Hg).

Menopause-related increases in blood pressure can be attributed in part to increased salt sensitivity (when too much sodium quickly leads to higher blood pressure, often triggering chronic high blood pressure) and weight gain. Both are associated with hormone changes during menopause.

Hormone therapy may be prescribed for a limited time after menopause to reduce postmenopausal symptoms, such as hot flashes and vaginal dryness. Those older than age 50 who take hormone therapy may have a small increase — usually 1 to 2 mm Hg — in systolic blood pressure.

Discuss the risks and benefits of hormone therapy with your health care team. Note that those who take hormone therapy respond to lifestyle changes and medications just as well as those who don't take hormone therapy.

BLACK, HISPANIC AND ASIAN PEOPLE

Studies examining the prevalence of high blood pressure in America show that the condition affects many more Black people than it does white people, Hispanic people and Asians. Hypertension in Black people also seems more likely to develop at a younger age and result in more severe complications than for those in other American ethnic groups.

Though the reasons for these differences are unclear, there are many theories. For example, research suggests that chronic stress related to a lifetime of discrimination is a factor. Nonetheless, the risk factors for hypertension — such as obesity, sleep apnea, physical inactivity, too much sodium and not enough potassium, excessive alcohol intake and not enough fruits and vegetables — are the same for everybody.

With proper medical care, the risk of stroke, heart attack and progressive

PULSE PRESSURE

Pulse pressure is the difference between the systolic and diastolic pressure readings. For example, if your systolic pressure is 120 mm Hg and your diastolic is 80 mm Hg, your pulse pressure is 40. This is considered a healthy pulse pressure.

Generally, a pulse pressure greater than 40 mm Hg is unhealthy. A pulse pressure greater than 60 is a risk factor for heart disease. A pulse pressure lower than 40 may mean you have poor heart function, while a higher pulse pressure may mean that your heart valves are leaky (valve regurgitation). Other conditions, including overactive thyroid (hyperthyroidism), can also increase pulse pressure.

kidney failure caused by high blood pressure can be reduced as effectively in Black people as in white people.

The use of diuretics, ACE inhibitors, ARBs and CCBs, alone or together, are effective treatments for Black individuals with hypertension. It's also important to note that Black participants in the DASH-Sodium study (see page 65) experienced the greatest reduction in their blood pressure. Black individuals also seem to benefit more than white individuals from increasing their potassium intake.

Rates of high blood pressure can vary among different ethnic groups. The prevalence of high blood pressure among some populations of American Indians is higher than in white people, for example. And among Hispanic people and Asians, the rate of high blood pressure is slightly lower than it is in whites.

OTHER CONDITIONS

Often, high blood pressure is accompanied by other medical conditions that make it more difficult to treat and control. If you have another chronic medical condition in addition to high blood pressure, it's especially critical that you see your health care team regularly. Several examples follow.

Cardiovascular problems

Cardiovascular conditions that often coexist with hypertension include:

Arrhythmia

High blood pressure can cause the heart to beat in an irregular rhythm. You're at greater risk of developing this condition if your blood contains low levels of potassium or magnesium, sometimes a result of treatment with diuretics. A high pulse pressure and thyroid disease will increase the risk, as well.

The most common arrhythmia is atrial fibrillation. Controlling high blood pressure decreases the amount of work the heart muscle has to do to pump blood. This, in turn, reduces the likelihood that you'll develop an arrhythmia.

To help control or prevent arrhythmia, with your health care team's consent, eat plenty of foods containing potassium and magnesium, such as fresh fruits and vegetables. If this doesn't help, you may need to take supplements to keep your potassium and magnesium levels at a healthy level. Eating fish high in omega-3 fatty acids or taking a fish oil supplement also may help lower your risk of sudden death as a result of arrhythmia. See Chapter 5 to learn more about fish oil supplements and types of fish to eat.

Arteriosclerosis and atherosclerosis

Over time, high pressure in the arteries can make the vessel walls thick and stiff, restricting blood flow. This is called arteriosclerosis (hardening of the arteries). Atherosclerosis is a specific type of arteriosclerosis caused by the buildup of fatty plaques in the walls of the arteries.

In addition to high blood pressure, risk factors include smoking, high levels of cholesterol and triglycerides, too much weight, lack of exercise, diabetes and excessive alcohol consumption. You may need to work on managing these factors.

In addition to controlling blood pressure, you may need to take medication to lower your cholesterol or triglycerides and blood sugar if they're too high, drink less alcohol, lose weight if you're overweight and get regular exercise.

Coronary artery disease

High blood pressure often coexists with coronary artery disease. Having high blood pressure puts added force against the walls of the arteries, which can damage the blood vessels and increase the risk of atherosclerosis. Atherosclerosis blocks blood vessels, including the coronary arteries — the heart's own circulatory system. Poor blood flow damages the heart muscle. This increases your risk of chest pain (angina), heart attack and heart failure.

Diuretics, beta blockers, ACE inhibitors, ARBs and aldosterone antagonists are often used to treat people with high blood pressure and coronary artery disease. That's because, in addition to lowering blood pressure, they reduce the risk of heart attack and heart failure. A beta blocker and calcium antagonist may be prescribed to relieve angina and, in some cases, reduce the risk of a second heart attack. Beta blockers have been shown to reduce plaques in coronary

arteries. In certain cases, surgical treatment of the coronary arteries, including angioplasty and the placement of stents, may be considered to keep the vessels open.

Your health care team may suggest daily aspirin therapy if you've already had a heart attack or stroke, or if you haven't had a heart attack but you have had a stent placed in a coronary artery, have had coronary bypass surgery or have chest pain due to coronary artery disease (angina).

Aspirin isn't recommended to prevent a heart attack in adults age 60 or older, but your health care team may consider it for you if you're between the ages of 40 and 59 and your risk is high of a heart-related event like a heart attack.

Heart failure

Heart failure can be the result of an enlarged, weakened heart, which has a hard time pumping enough blood to meet the body's needs. Or the heart might pump OK, but a thickening of the pumping chamber on the left side of the heart doesn't allow the muscle to expand and relax as it should (diastolic heart failure). In some cases, this can cause fluid to build up in the lungs or the feet and legs.

Lowering blood pressure helps the heart not have to work as hard. In fact, the most remarkable benefit of well-controlled high blood pressure is that it can lower the risk of developing heart failure by more than half.

ACE inhibitors, ARBs and diuretics may be prescribed if you have heart failure and high blood pressure. ACE inhibitors and ARBs reduce blood pressure by opening (dilating) the blood vessels, without interfering with the heart's pumping action.

Diuretics reduce fluid buildup. The potassium-sparing diuretics spironolactone (Aldactone) and eplerenone (Inspra), which block aldosterone, can offer lifesaving benefits for people with heart failure.

In most cases, a beta blocker also may be appropriate. If you don't tolerate ACE inhibitors, your health care team may prescribe an alternative, such as an ARB. Depending on your circumstances, you may choose to see a heart failure specialist, because treatment programs for heart failure are complex and a heart transplant may need to be considered.

High cholesterol

Many people with high blood pressure also have high cholesterol. Because having both conditions increases the risk of heart attack and stroke, there are benefits from lowering both cholesterol and blood pressure. The same lifestyle changes that help lower blood pressure can help lower cholesterol levels. However, many people with high cholesterol also need a cholesterol-lowering drugs.

High doses of high blood pressure medications can increase cholesterol and triglyceride levels. Low doses of these drugs don't produce the same effects. Beta blockers also may slightly raise cholesterol. If you need to take high doses of a beta blocker, a healthy diet and cholesterol-lowering drugs can help counteract the increase.

If you're taking cholesterol-lowering medication, it's important to avoid eating Seville (sour) oranges, pomelos or grapefruit, and drinking grapefruit juices. An interaction between the juice of these fruits and the statin can lead to a drug buildup in the blood. The same is true for some calcium channel blockers, so ask your health care team what's best.

Metabolic syndrome

Metabolic syndrome is a cluster of conditions that occur together and increase the risk of heart disease, stroke and type 2 diabetes. These conditions include increased blood pressure, high blood sugar, too much fat around the waist and high cholesterol or triglyceride levels.

Having just one of these conditions increases the risk of heart disease, stroke and diabetes. But in combination, risk is even greater. Many people with metabolic syndrome may also have sleep apnea.

Research into understanding the complex processes that form this syndrome is ongoing. Many believe it's caused by a mix of genetic and environmental factors, including insulin resistance, abdominal obesity, genetics, elevated blood pressure and chronic stress.

The different components of metabolic syndrome are generally treated at the same time to reduce risk. Exercising regularly, losing weight, quitting smoking and reducing intake of sodium, sugar, saturated fat and trans fats help improve all aspects of metabolic syndrome, including lowering blood pressure and reducing cholesterol and blood sugar levels.

If lifestyle modifications aren't enough, you may need to take medications to lower blood pressure, control cholesterol or promote weight loss. Insulin sensitizers may help your body use insulin more effectively.

Diabetes

Diabetes and high blood pressure are closely linked. According to the American Diabetes Association, about two-thirds of adults with diabetes report having high blood pressure and, conversely, people with untreated high blood pressure have a higher rate of diabetes. Having both conditions is a serious concern.

Many of the complications associated with diabetes can be attributed to having high blood pressure. A combination of high blood pressure, diabetes, high cholesterol and tobacco use puts you at extremely high risk of a heart attack.

Aim to achieve optimal blood pressure, blood sugar (glucose) and blood fats. Aim to lower your blood pressure to 130/80 mm Hg or lower if possible. If you also have kidney disease, you may need to strive for an even lower goal. Talk to your health care team about the blood pressure goal that makes the most sense for you.

Lifestyle changes can help reduce the risk of serious complications from both diabetes and high blood pressure: Eat a healthy diet, get regular exercise, limit alcohol, and if you smoke or chew tobacco, stop doing so.

People who also have high cholesterol respond well to aggressive management. Lifestyle changes can reduce the risk of developing diabetes by half if you have prediabetes, impaired fasting glucose or obesity.

Medical therapy usually consists of ACE inhibitors or ARBs. They help protect the kidneys, which are more likely to be damaged if you have both diabetes and high blood pressure. These drugs also have relatively few side effects.

Diuretics, beta blockers and calcium channel blockers also may be used to lower blood pressure and to prolong life. Alpha blockers are generally recommended last because they may worsen orthostatic hypotension, a problem in some people with diabetes, and increase the risk of heart failure.

Often, combination drug therapy is needed to reach the target goal. If you're taking diuretics, your health care team will aim to keep your blood levels of potassium in a healthy range through diet or supplements to reduce the likelihood of new-onset diabetes.

Sleep apnea

Obstructive sleep apnea is a disorder in which breathing stops and starts repeatedly during sleep. It's relatively common in people with high blood pressure, particularly when it's difficult to control. Daytime drowsiness, snoring and prolonged pauses in breathing while sleeping are clues that the condition may be present.

Other symptoms include waking with a dry mouth, morning headache, gasping for air during sleep, not sleeping well, trouble paying attention while awake and feeling irritable. Obstructed airways, as well as disturbances in the way the brain controls breathing, can cause sleep apnea. Obstructive sleep apnea can increase the risk of heart attack, stroke, and heart arrhythmias such as atrial fibrillation.

Although obesity is a risk factor for both hypertension and sleep apnea, recent studies suggest that sleep apnea helps lead to hypertension, whether a person is overweight or not.

One theory centers on the fact that when breathing stops during sleep, these pauses activate sympathetic nerve pathways, the part of the nervous system that prepares the body to react to stress or danger. Activating this system raises blood pressure.

Sleep apnea is also associated with frequent arousals in brain activity, after which breathing resumes. The exaggerated activation of the sympathetic drive even during wakefulness — which occurs in people with sleep apnea — may result in a sustained increase in blood pressure.

More studies need to be done on the relationship between sleep apnea and hypertension. It's likely that treating sleep apnea — with continuous positive airway pressure (CPAP) therapy, weight loss and regular exercise — will improve daytime and nighttime blood pressure and decrease the risk of cardiovascular disease.

Kidney disease

The kidneys play a vital role in removing extra fluid and waste from the body. This helps keep blood pressure under control. But if the blood vessels in the kidneys are damaged from high blood pressure, the organs may become less efficient. This allows excess fluid to remain in the circulatory system, making high blood pressure worse. In turn, high blood pressure further weakens kidneys.

Most people with chronic kidney disease also have high blood pressure. The more impaired the kidneys are, the greater the risk of coronary artery disease, a common cause of disability and death among people who have chronic kidney disease.

Eventually, high blood pressure can lead to kidney (renal) failure, a condition in which the kidneys no longer function. In this end stage, life must be sustained with kidney dialysis or a kidney transplant.

If you have kidney and heart disease because of high blood pressure, you'll need to take medications and make lifestyle changes to prevent further damage to your kidneys and cardiovascular system. Black individuals in America are more likely than are white individuals to develop kidney problems from high blood pressure. Identifying and treating hypertension early is the best option for preventing kidney problems from ever occurring.

Once your blood pressure is lowered, the decline in kidney function also slows. If you have advanced kidney failure, you'll likely have special dietary needs that are best discussed with a dietitian. For example, reducing sodium in your diet is important because impaired kidney function increases the level of sodium and fluids in your body.

Choice of blood pressure medication is also important. ACE inhibitors and ARBs are often the best medications for preventing further damage to the kidneys, and may be combined with a diuretic. However, these medications need to be used with caution because of potential side effects, such as too much potassium in the blood (hyperkalemia). Several drugs are usually needed to reach a blood pressure goal.

A potentially reversible cause of kidney failure is the narrowing of the main artery leading to one or both kidneys. Atherosclerosis is the most common cause. Your health care team may consider widening the narrowed artery with procedures such as angioplasty, stenting or surgery if aggressive drug therapy doesn't help.

Sexual dysfunction

Some evidence shows a higher rate of sexual dysfunction in people who have high blood pressure. Erectile dysfunction (impotence, or ED) is more likely in men with untreated high blood pressure than in those who take medication. Other risk factors are similar to those for heart disease and include diabetes, high blood fats, obesity and lack of physical activity.

How high blood pressure affects sexual function isn't well understood, but it's possible for high blood pressure to affect your sex life. High blood pressure can reduce blood flow to the vagina. For some, this leads to a decrease in sexual desire or arousal, vaginal dryness or difficulty achieving orgasm. Finding effective methods of arousal and using lubrication can help.

Anyone can experience anxiety and relationship issues due to sexual dysfunction. That's why it's important to talk about sexual difficulties with a health care provider.

How high blood pressure and the medications used to treat it affect sexual function in men is a topic that's received significant attention. Research shows that among frequently used blood pressure medications, thiazide diuretics and beta blockers — especially nonselective types of beta blockers — have been linked to sexual dysfunction in men.

If you experience problems related to sexual dysfunction, you may be able to take a different blood pressure medication

- Women have specific issues related to high blood pressure that merit special attention.
- High blood pressure during pregnancy must be monitored closely because of the risk to the mother and to the baby if left untreated.
- High blood pressure in Black people appears to develop at a younger age and result in more severe complications than in most other American ethnic groups.
- Aggressive treatment is necessary when high blood pressure is associated with another condition such as diabetes, high cholesterol, cardiovascular disease, stroke or kidney disease.
- Don't settle for poorly controlled hypertension. Work with your health care team to achieve your treatment goals.

that's less likely to affect sexual function. ACE inhibitors, alpha blockers, calcium channel blockers and ARBs are all options. In addition, another class of drugs is available for men who experience erectile dysfunction. It includes the drugs sildenafil (Viagra), tadalafil (Cialis) and vardenafil (Levitra, Staxyn). Ask your health care team if these medications might be appropriate for you.

Before starting a high blood pressure medication, don't hesitate to discuss your current sexual function with your health care team. Also, once you start taking a high blood pressure medication, be sure to report any changes you experience.

Living well with high blood pressure

10

High blood pressure isn't an illness you can treat and then ignore. It's a chronic health condition, something you'll need to manage for the rest of your life. The good news is that you can develop an effective plan to manage your high blood pressure with your health care team.

Sometimes, staying motivated to manage high blood pressure can be difficult because you typically can't feel or see that anything is wrong. With many health conditions, such as arthritis or allergies, the symptoms you experience motivate you to treat the condition. You feel the flaring pain and stiffness of arthritic joints, or you experience the sneezing and itchy eyes of an allergy attack. You're motivated to take care of the condition because you want those bothersome signs and symptoms to go away. But high blood pressure is different.

The lack of symptoms is one of many reasons people with high blood pressure often don't take proper steps to manage it. It's also part of the reason why only about half of Americans with high blood pressure have it under control.

Others may pretend that they have little to worry about. Despite good advice from their health care providers, they go about their everyday lives, and whether or not they stick to their treatment programs seems to make little difference — until organ damage and serious complications occur. That's why high blood pressure is often called the "silent killer."

Actively taking part in your health care and managing your blood pressure — measuring it at home, taking medications properly, eating a healthy diet, getting regular physical activity, seeing your health care team regularly — are essential. These efforts can significantly boost your chances of living a longer, healthier life, despite high blood pressure.

There are many steps you can take to successfully manage high blood pressure. Here's more on what you can do.

HOW ARE YOUR OTHER BEHAVIORS?

1. Do you smoke cigarettes, cigars or pipes or use snuff or chewing tobacco?
   - ☐ Yes (1 point)
   - ☐ Very infrequently (2 points)
   - ☐ No (3 points)

2. Do you drink more than a moderate amount of alcohol? (A moderate amount is one drink a day for women and for men age 65 and older, and two drinks a day for men younger than 65.)
   - ☐ Yes or quite often (1 point)
   - ☐ Sometimes (2 points)
   - ☐ Never or infrequently (3 points)

3. Do you see a health care provider for regular checkups?
   - ☐ No (1 point)
   - ☐ Sometimes (2 points)
   - ☐ Yes (3 points)

4. Do you wake up multiple times during the night or snore while you're asleep?
   - ☐ Often (1 point)
   - ☐ Occasionally (2 points)
   - ☐ Never or infrequently (3 points)

5. Do you often feel sleepy during the day and have trouble functioning because you're tired?
   - ☐ Often (1 point)
   - ☐ Occasionally (2 points)
   - ☐ Never or infrequently (3 points)

MANAGE STRESS

If you lead a stressful life, you'll have high blood pressure, right? This commonly held belief isn't entirely true. Many people have high stress and don't have high blood pressure, just as many laid-back people have high blood pressure.

It's true that when you're anxious or under a tight deadline, your blood pressure may increase. Then as you relax, your blood pressure generally returns to its usual level. But chronic stress, in situations that aren't short-lived, may help lead to high blood pressure. Studies show that people who are characteristically

6. How would you rate your ability to manage daily stress?
   - ☐ Poor (1 point)
   - ☐ Fair (2 points)
   - ☐ Good (3 points)

7. How often do you feel lonely, depressed or pessimistic about what's happening around you?
   - ☐ Often or always (1 point)
   - ☐ Occasionally (2 points)
   - ☐ Never or infrequently (3 points)

»» How did you score?

To the right of the answer you chose is a point value — 1, 2 or 3 points. Add up the points from your answers for your total score.

A: If your total score was 18 to 21 points, congratulations! You're making wise decisions regarding your health.

B: If your score was 13 to 17 points, you're on the right track, but there's room for improvement.

C: If your score was 7 to 12 points, your behaviors may be putting your health in jeopardy. Select areas where you can try to make improvements.

impatient or hostile — traits commonly associated with stress — are more likely to develop high blood pressure.

If you have high blood pressure, managing stress may not lower your blood pressure to your goal, but managing stress is important for other reasons:

- **Better long-term control.** Even temporary increases in blood pressure caused by stress can make high blood pressure more difficult to manage. If you're able to effectively manage your stress, you may have a better chance of keeping your blood pressure lower.
- **More positive attitude.** Stress can erode your commitment and motivation to control your high blood pressure. It's much easier to be physically active, eat a healthy diet, lose weight and limit alcohol when you're less stressed.

There are many ways to manage stress. By experimenting with different approaches and techniques, you'll find the stress management strategies that fit your lifestyle and daily routine.

What is stress?

Think of stress as a spice. Too little spice results in a bland-tasting meal. Too much spice can muddle flavors or make the food inedible. With the right amount, spice can provide a memorable eating experience.

Stress works in the same way on your health and well-being. You need some stress to keep your life interesting and challenging, but too much stress can overwhelm you. The issue is finding the right balance.

Stress is a natural part of daily life. It's what you experience when you deal with demands that cause you to feel some degree of emotional or physical pressure that challenges your ability to cope. Stress is not the demands themselves (known as stressors) but rather how you respond to them.

Stress can provide feelings of excitement, opportunity and accomplishment. This is known as positive stress. In these circumstances, you feel confident and motivated. Positive stress often drives athletes to perform well in competition.

Other examples of positive stress may include working toward a college degree, getting married, starting a new job and experiencing childbirth.

But stress can also make you feel out of control or overwhelmed. This is negative stress. You may have trouble staying focused on the task at hand or feel isolated and picked on by others. Family relationships, financial problems, work deadlines and poor health are common sources of negative stress. Stress becomes negative when you face continuous challenges without relief or relaxation between challenges.

Physiologically, your body tends to respond to any stressful challenge in the same way. How you see that challenge is what makes the stress positive or negative for you.

That's what makes stress vary from person to person. What may be stressful for you may not be stressful for someone else. Some people generally cope well with difficult or tense situations, while others experience a high level of perceived stress. For many reasons, someone who managed stress well one week may have trouble coping with a similar kind of stress the following week.

What happens when you face stress?

Racing against a deadline, being stuck in traffic, arguing with a spouse — these intense situations can make the body react as though it were facing a physical threat.

The stress response, often referred to as the fight-or-flight response, switches the body into high gear. It provides the energy, speed and focus either to meet the challenge head-on (fight) or to get out of the way (flight).

The fight-or-flight response can occur during any situation that's seen as dangerous, even if it's not. Your view of a threat can cause a surge of hormones that shifts your body into overdrive. Among the hormones are epinephrine (adrenaline) and cortisol, which cause your heart to beat faster and your blood pressure to increase. Other physical changes also occur. Breathing quickens, blood sugar rises and more blood and nutrients are sent to the brain and large muscles.

WARNING SIGNS OF STRESS

Some of the most common signs and symptoms of stress include:
- Frequently feeling stressed out
- Overwhelming feelings of anger, frustration or anxiety
- Frequent headaches, backaches or colds
- Insomnia or other sleep disorders
- Increased use of alcohol or medications
- Feelings of grief, hopelessness or depression
- Less of a sense of humor
- Loss of interest in usual activities
- Periods of crying or other emotional outbursts
- Lack of attention to physical health and appearance
- Unhealthy eating, such as binge eating or snacking on junk food

Just because you don't have any of these signs and symptoms doesn't mean that you're not under stress. You may not recognize the signs.

The nervous system also springs into action. The pupils of the eyes widen (dilate) to boost vision. Facial muscles tense up to make you look more intimidating. Sweating cools the body.

Too much stress can change behavior, too. You may become easily discouraged, irritable, cynical, emotional or even reclusive. All these feelings affect how you think and act. However, these changes are sometimes easy to miss because they develop little by little over time.

Physical signs and symptoms of stress aren't as easy to ignore. They may include headache, stomach upset, insomnia, fatigue and frequent illness. You may revert to nervous habits, such as biting your nails or smoking.

The hormones epinephrine and cortisol are released during periods of high stress. They increase blood pressure by narrowing blood vessels and increasing heart rate. The increase in blood pressure varies depending on how intense the stressor is and on how the body copes with the challenge. In some people, stress causes only a slight increase in blood pressure. In others, it can produce extreme jumps.

The effects of stress on the body are usually only temporary. However, if you regularly experience high levels of stress, over time these increases can gradually damage the arteries, heart, brain, kidneys and eyes. Taken together, these effects of stress often go unrecognized until the condition manifests itself as persistent high blood pressure.

Steps to soothe stress

Stress can come from many sources: relationships, work, family or deadlines. Turn to these tools to stay on track during stressful times.

Mindfulness

Mindfulness is the act of being intensely aware of what you're sensing and feeling at the present moment — without interpretation or judgment. Mindfulness involves maintaining a moment-to-moment awareness of where you are and what you're doing. At work, for instance, it means you're focused on the project in front of you, not thinking about future deadlines. If you're walking with a friend, it gives you the ability to really focus on your surroundings and your conversation.

Researchers have shown that you can train your brain to become more mindful. It just takes practice.

Mindfulness-based stress reduction (MBSR) training has become a recognized way to help people learn to avoid distractions and increase their attention to the task in front of them. MBSR programs typically include breathing, stretching and awareness exercises.

Look for times in your day where you can focus your attention, such as mindfully eating your dinner by engaging your senses to notice the taste, aromas and textures of each dish. Or try focusing on your breath, noticing the coolness of the air as you inhale and the warmth as you exhale. Can you feel the rise and fall of your chest with each breath?

You'll likely be surprised by what you notice when you simply take the time to pay attention. And as you become more aware of your world, you might become fonder of the things around you, which brings comfort, not stress.

Mindful movement

The hallmarks of yoga — structured breathing, controlled movement, mental focus — are the perfect antidote to stress and distracted thinking.

Many studies have found that, after beginning a yoga program, people feel less stressed, more focused, even more optimistic. In fact, yoga's been found to be even more beneficial to people who are highly stressed.

There are other ways to be mindful during physical activity, too.

For example, during structured physical activity such as a brisk walk, try to be mindful by paying attention to the details around you. Or when you're playing golf, practice mindfulness by focusing on every moment of your game instead of letting your mind wander to work or things you need to do at home.

Gratitude

Focusing on what you're grateful for each day has been shown to significantly

STRESS AND YOUR HEALTH

Stress is thought to play a role in several medical conditions. When heart rate increases, the risks of chest pain (angina) and irregularities in heart rhythm (arrhythmia) are higher. Stress-related surges in heart rate and blood pressure also can trigger a heart attack or damage the heart muscle or coronary arteries. The blood-clotting protein fibrin, which is released when you're under stress, also puts you at increased risk of blood clots.

The hormone cortisol is released during stress, and it may suppress the immune system. There's evidence that this suppression may make it more likely you'll catch an infectious disease, including upper respiratory viral infections such as cold or flu. Stress also can trigger headaches and may worsen asthma and intestinal problems. It may also slow wound healing. Use this awareness of the connections between stress and health as motivation to find ways to manage your stress effectively.

increase happiness — and physical health. In addition to improving sleep, practicing gratitude can boost immunity, decrease risk of disease and reduce stress.

Here are a few tips to get started:

Write in a gratitude journal. Write in a journal every day. Keep a daily log of three things you're grateful for. They can be as simple as something funny one of your children did or a kind gesture from a stranger at the grocery store. Any positive thoughts or actions count, no matter how small.

Use gratitude cues. Any new habit needs reminders. Cues are a great way to stay on course. Keep in front of you pictures of things or people that make you happy. Post positive notes or inspirational quotes on the fridge or by your computer to reinforce feelings of gratitude.

Keep a gratitude jar. Keep an empty jar, scratch paper and a pen in an accessible

HOW DO I STAY IN CONTROL OF STRESSFUL SITUATIONS?

When you're trying to manage stress, consider one of these four As when you're looking for a solution:

Avoid
A lot of needless stress can simply be avoided. Don't like traffic jams? Leave for work early. Hate waiting in line at the cafeteria? Pack a lunch. When you can, avoid negative people.

Alter
Try to change your situation so things will have a chance to work better in the future. Respectfully talk with others about their behaviors and be willing to change your behavior if needed. Manage your time better.

Adapt
Changing your standards or expectations is one of the best ways to deal with stress. Look at your situation from a new perspective. Think more about the positives in life and less about the negatives. Focus on the big picture.

Accept
If you have no choice but to accept things as they are, try to forgive. Talk to a friend. Learn from your mistakes. And be grateful for the positive things in your life.

place at home. Each day write down on a piece of paper one thing that you're grateful for and drop it in the jar. Encourage your family members to do the same. During dinner or when you have some time, take a few of the notes out of the jar and enjoy reading one another's thoughts.

The goal is to move your mind from thinking about gratitude occasionally to feeling grateful on a daily basis.

Meditation

Meditation aims to increase your awareness of the present moment and help you develop a gentle, accepting attitude toward yourself. Regular meditation practice has been shown to alter the brain — in a good way.

When you meditate, you focus attention on your breathing or on repeating a word, phrase, image or sound to clear your mind of distracting thoughts. Most types of meditation require four elements: a quiet place; relaxed posture; focused attention; and an open attitude in which distractions come and go and you gently bring your attention back to the focus.

Meditation can lead to a state of physical relaxation and psychological balance. It's also been shown to affect your body's stress reaction.

One study showed that the area of the brain dedicated to regulating your emotions was significantly larger in people who were experienced meditators. In other words, in a world determined to

trip you up with distractions and unpleasant surprises, meditation can help you stay more positive and more focused.

Guided imagery

Also known as visualization, this method of relaxation relies on memories or images to view with your mind's eye. You experience a peaceful setting with all your senses, as if you were actually there, imagining the sounds, scents, colors and tactile sensations. The messages your brain receives from this imagery help your body relax.

Relaxed breathing

Stress typically causes rapid, shallow breathing from your chest, which sustains other aspects of the stress reaction, such as rapid heart rate and perspiration. You breathe correctly when you breathe deeply from your diaphragm, and your belly — not only your chest — moves with each breath.

Deep, slow breathing from your diaphragm is a powerful and simple strategy for blood pressure control. Plus, it's relaxing. Deep breathing acts on centers in the brain that lower blood pressure. If you're able to control shallow breathing and to relax, the effects of acute stress will decrease (see page 158).

A medical device called Resperate is designed to help lower blood pressure with deep breathing. The device includes a respiration sensor, headphones and a small unit that looks like a portable CD player.

Resperate analyzes your breathing pattern and creates two distinct melodic tones to guide your inhalation and exhalation. If you're synchronized to the melody, you can slow your breathing to fewer than 10 breaths a minute. To achieve a lasting reduction in systolic pressure, you'll need to use Resperate for about 15 minutes a day, three or four days a week. Within a few weeks, these exercises may help lower blood pressure.

Research involving this device indicates that slow breathing can cause a small but significant decrease in blood pressure in some people. It's unclear how long the effects last, or if continued use lowers blood pressure even more. But slow breathing is easy to do and costs nothing, and there are few, if any, side effects.

Muscle tension exercises

Tension and stress can cause muscles to tighten, especially in the shoulders and

TAKE A BREATHER

Here's an exercise to help you practice relaxed breathing.

1.   Wear comfortable clothes that are loose around your waist. You may lie on your back or sit in a comfortable chair, whichever you prefer.
2.   Lie or sit with your feet slightly apart, with one hand resting on your belly and the other hand on your chest. If you're sitting, place your feet flat on the floor, relax your shoulders and place your hands in your lap or at your side.
3.   Inhale through your nose, if you can, because this filters and warms the air. Exhale through your mouth.
4.   Focus on your breathing for a few minutes. Then gently exhale most of the air in your lungs.
5.   Inhale while slowly counting to four, about one second per count. As you inhale, slightly raise your belly, about 1 inch. You should be able to feel the movement with your hand.
6.   As you breathe in, imagine the air flowing to all parts of your body, supplying you with cleansing, energizing oxygen.
7.   Pause for a second with the air in your lungs. Then slowly exhale, counting to four. You'll feel your belly slowly fall as your diaphragm relaxes. Imagine the tension flowing out of you.
8.   Pause for a moment. Then repeat this exercise for 1 to 2 minutes, until you feel better. If you experience lightheadedness, shorten the length or depth of your breathing.

neck. To relieve the tightness, roll your shoulders, raising them toward your ears. Then relax your shoulders and neck.

To further reduce neck tension, gently move your head clockwise in a circle, then counterclockwise. To relieve tension in your back and torso, reach toward the ceiling and do side bends. For foot and leg tension, draw circles in the air with your feet while flexing your toes.

Progressive muscle relaxation can help reduce tension, anxiety and stress. Starting with your feet and working up through your body to your head and neck, tense each muscle group for at least five seconds and then relax the muscles for up to 30 seconds. Repeat before moving to the next muscle group.

Adopt a positive outlook

Studies suggest that an optimistic attitude helps you to cope better with stressful situations, likely reducing the effects stress has on the body. So it's not surprising that a pessimistic outlook can make it much harder to deal with even minor stressors. Here are ways you can improve your outlook on life.

Monitor self-talk

The endless stream of thoughts that run through your head can be positive or negative. You can reduce stress by learning how to reframe negative thoughts and practice positive thinking. For example, instead of telling yourself, "I should never make a mistake because I'll look stupid," try thinking, "Everyone makes mistakes. I will learn from this experience." This approach can lead to a more realistic and self-affirming outlook.

Manage anger

Everyday frustrations can cause your temper to flare. But if your blood boils after even minor irritations or you're constantly seething, you may need to work at getting your anger under control. Anger that's out of control is destructive. It can lead to problems in your relationships, health and enjoyment of life.

How can you control anger? Think carefully before saying something you'll later regret. Count to 10 before reacting or leave the situation if you can. Find ways to calm and soothe yourself. When ready, express your anger in a controlled and appropriate manner that respects the rights of others so that you aren't left stewing. And avoid holding grudges.

Look for humor

Laughter is a natural high: It doesn't just lighten your load mentally; it actually induces physical reactions in the body. When you laugh, your heart, lungs and muscles are stimulated. Laughter also releases chemicals in your brain called endorphins that ease pain and enhance a feeling of well-being. If you use humor to deal with setbacks positively, you're more likely to take a positive approach.

Schedule worry time

If you're facing a challenging situation, setting aside a specific time for problem-solving can help keep worries from building up inside you or keeping you awake at night.

Devote time each day to work on solutions to problems that are causing stress and assess your progress in solving them. If a worry crops up outside of worry time, write it down and tell yourself you will worry about it during your scheduled worry time. Be sure to plan a positive activity to engage in after your worry time.

Adapt your lifestyle

Making healthy changes to your daily routine also can help you manage stress. Plus, a healthy lifestyle is good for your overall health. Eating well, moving more and getting enough sleep are all helpful, but there's more you can do to improve your lifestyle.

Get plenty of sleep

Studies show that people who have poor sleep quality are more likely to develop hypertension. Poor sleep quality includes chronic insomnia, reduced sleep duration and disrupted sleep. Sleep apnea can cause and aggravate high blood pressure. (See page 146 for more on sleep apnea.)

When you're refreshed from a good night's sleep, you're better able to manage the stressors that come your way the next day. Going to bed and waking at consistent times each day can help you sleep better. Slow the pace of evening activities to establish a calming environment. A bedtime routine can aid in falling asleep.

Move more

Physical activity is a fantastic way to manage stress. Add at least 10 minutes of moderate physical activity to what you already do every day. Adding just this much physical activity makes a difference. Did you know that just 60 to 90 minutes a week of physical activity can reduce your heart disease risk by up to half? That's a big benefit from a pretty small commitment on your part.

It doesn't have to be major. Take the stairs, take a walk — just get moving. As you become more active, work toward increasing your total amount of physical activity every day.

Eat well

Stress can trigger overeating episodes. Many people turn to high-calorie, high-fat comfort food when they're dealing with a difficult problem or are at a weak emotional point. When this urge strikes, try to distract yourself by calling a friend or going for a walk. When your mind is occupied with something positive, the urge for overeating can quickly go away.

A healthy approach to eating includes a wide variety of foods that taste good and are good for you. Eat more vegetables, fruits and whole grains, which are packed with nutrition generally low in calories. These foods contain antioxidants, dietary fiber and other disease-fighting substances that help keep your body systems in good working order.

Get organized

Prepare a written schedule of weekly activities, highlighting priority tasks. Being organized will help reduce time conflicts, missed appointments and last-minute deadlines. Schedule important tasks — especially those that seem most stressful — at the time of day when you're feeling your best.

Simplify your schedule

Try to adopt a more relaxed pace. Assess your time commitments, and don't feel obligated or guilty if you say no to requests or social invitations that you know you can't handle. Look to others for help or delegate responsibilities.

Relieve work-related stress

Job frustration can be a major source of stress. To relieve worry and disappointment, take time to do high-quality work but don't strive for perfection. Show respect for others and a willingness to resolve conflicts with coworkers. Identify skills you'll need for your long-term career goals and create a plan for developing those skills.

Build a financial cushion

Try to put part of every paycheck in a savings account or low-risk investment. Having reserve funds in the bank is one way to cope with unexpected financial stress such as the loss of a job, a salary cut or a large, unplanned-for expense. Even if an emergency use for the money never arrives, just knowing that you have a financial cushion can reduce stress.

Stand tall

Observe your posture when you feel overly stressed. You may find that you slump your shoulders, your breathing becomes shallow and you're less active. Stress may cause you to neglect your appearance.

Good posture helps relieve aches and pains by placing less strain on your muscles and allowing you to move efficiently. To promote good posture, stand with your weight on both feet, shoulders back and stomach muscles tight. Keep your back well supported when you're seated.

Take occasional breaks

When you're feeling stressed, do you find yourself working through all of your breaks? There's a better way.

Take opportunities to stretch, walk and relax during your regular day. Use brief vacations, even if they're just for a day or the weekend, to allow yourself time away from stressful environments. Pursue hobbies and recreational activities that you enjoy. Quality leisure time reduces stress and improves your outlook on life.

Maintain social relationships

In times of high stress, it's common to isolate yourself from others. But friends and family can provide a valuable release valve when you need to vent your emotions. They can also give you encouragement and helpful advice. However, avoid confiding in people who tend to be negative about everything and who foster bad feelings. Surround yourself with supportive people.

Seek help if you need it

Sometimes, life's problems pile up and may become more than you can deal with on your own. If you feel overwhelmed by stress, consider getting help from your health care team or from a licensed mental health provider. Some people believe that seeking outside help is a sign of personal weakness. Nothing could be further from the truth. It takes strength of character to admit that you need help and to seek it.

Learning how to control stress won't guarantee you'll have a normal blood pressure, let alone a relaxed life and good health. Unexpected stressors will still occur. But having the tools to cope with stress can make those challenges easier to overcome — and your blood pressure easier to control.

TAKE YOUR BLOOD PRESSURE AT HOME

A medical office isn't the only place to measure blood pressure. The American Heart Association and other medical organizations recommend all individuals with high blood pressure monitor their blood pressure at home. Home monitoring allows you to track your blood pressure during your daily routine and in circumstances separate from a medical office or hospital visit.

The information you compile from home monitoring is vital to your blood pressure treatment program. It can help your health care team determine if the prescribed treatment of your condition is working and if adjustments need to be made.

If your blood pressure is well controlled, you may only need to check it at home a few days each month. Take two readings in the morning and two in the evening on a day that you're working and two pairs of readings on a day that you're relaxing.

If you're just starting home monitoring, if you're making changes to your medications or if you have other health conditions, you may need to check it more often — perhaps daily.

How to do it

Here's how to take your blood pressure to receive the most accurate results. Ask your health care team for additional instructions if needed.

Step 1

Measure your blood pressure at the same time each day, such as morning or evening or both, based on the recommendation of your health care team.

Be consistent with which arm you use. If you're right-handed, you may find it easier to measure pressure in your left arm and vice versa. But first, check the instructions that came with your device to make sure that it will sense your blood pressure with either arm. Also, confirm with your health care team which arm you should use.

Step 2

Approximately 30 minutes before you take your blood pressure, don't smoke, drink a caffeinated beverage or exercise. Five minutes before the measurement, sit still in a quiet place.

Step 3

Stretch out your arm, palm upward. Place the cuff on your bare upper arm one inch above the bend of your elbow. (It's important that the cuff is the right size for your arm.) You know that the sensor is correctly placed if the tubing falls over the front center of your arm. Pull the end of the cuff so that it's evenly tight around your arm. You want it tight enough so that you can only slip two fingertips under the top edge of the cuff. Make sure your skin doesn't pinch when the cuff inflates.

Step 4

Rest your cuffed arm on a flat surface, like a table, and have it at the level of your heart — not too high or too low. Sit upright with your back straight and supported and both feet flat on the floor.

Step 5

Start the machine. The cuff will inflate and then slowly deflate to take your measurement. Don't talk during this time and remain still and quiet. When the reading is complete, the monitor will display your blood pressure on the digital panel.

Step 6

Once you've taken your blood pressure, wait 1 to 3 minutes and do it again. Blood pressure can vary as much as 5 to 10 millimeters of mercury during a breathing cycle. So don't expect the readings to be the same. But if the readings vary widely, consider taking a third measurement and averaging the three.

In a log or journal or on a printable online tracker, jot down the average of the two readings. Find a sample log you can use on page 168.

Step 7

Bring your blood pressure readings with you to your next checkup. If you have a monitor with built-in memory that stores

Using an electronic model involves sitting with your arm at heart level, placing the cuff around your upper arm, relaxing and pressing a button to inflate the cuff and get a reading.

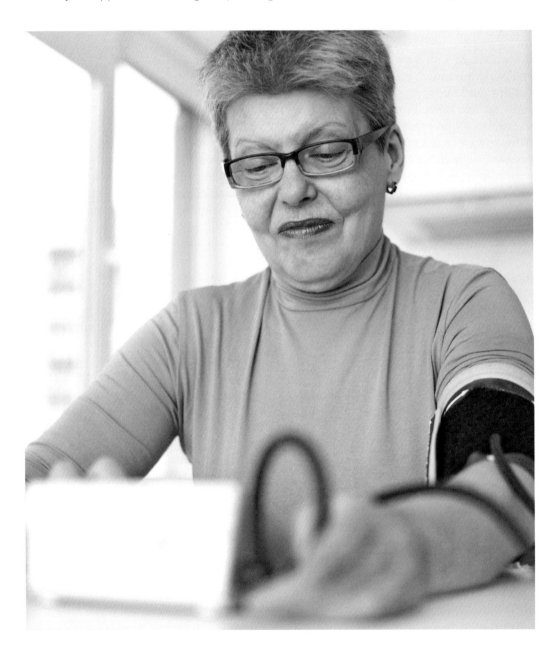

the results, bring the monitor to your checkup. Some monitors are equipped so they can upload your blood pressure readings automatically into a computer or mobile device or send them electronically to your health care team.

Step 8

If you have trouble getting consistent readings, check with your health care team. The problem may be your technique or your equipment. To see a video demonstration of how to use an electron-ic home blood pressure monitor, visit www.MayoClinic.org and search for "How to measure blood pressure using an automatic monitor."

Contact your health care team if you notice an unusual or persistent increase in your blood pressure.

Types of blood pressure monitors

Not all blood pressure monitors are the same. Some are easier to use, some are more reliable and some are inaccurate.

ELECTRONIC MONITOR

Electronic blood pressure monitors include a digital gauge and cuff that inflates at the push of a button.

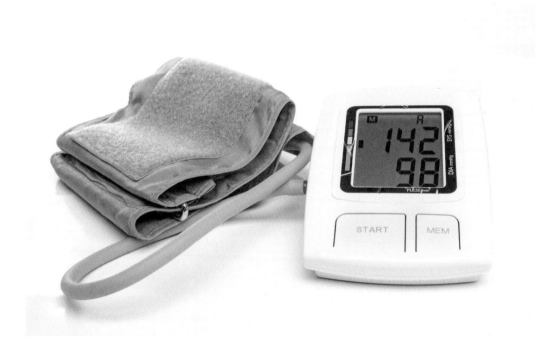

When buying a blood pressure monitor, consider these factors:

Cuff size

A properly fitting cuff is the most important factor to consider. A cuff that doesn't fit properly won't give an accurate blood pressure measurement. Ask your health care team what cuff size you need. Ideally, the cuff will have a D-ring fastener to securely close it.

Display

The display that shows your blood pressure measurement should be clear and easy to read.

Cost

Prices vary. Ask your health insurance provider if your policy covers the cost of a home blood pressure monitor.

After you buy a home monitor, bring it to your next appointment so your health care team can make sure you're using it correctly. Then, once a year, take it with you to an appointment so it can be tested to make sure its readings are accurate.

Automatic models

Also referred to as digital electronic blood pressure monitors, these models are the most popular and easiest to use for home monitoring. They also tend to be more expensive than older manual devices, though the cost continues to decline.

Automatic blood pressure monitors detect motion in the artery wall rather than the sound of blood flow.

These types of blood pressure monitors generally require you to do two things — properly wrap the inflatable cuff around your arm and push a button with your finger. The cuff automatically inflates with air and then slowly deflates. Your blood pressure is displayed on the digital gauge.

If you need a large-size adult cuff, several automatic monitors come with both regular and large cuffs or a choice between the two sizes when you purchase them.

If you have an irregular heart rhythm, check with your health care team before you buy an automatic model — it may not give you an accurate reading. Some newer digital units can sense an irregular pulse accurately. This feature is generally listed on the unit's packaging.

Finger or wrist models

To make blood pressure monitors smaller and easy to use, some manufacturers have developed models that measure blood pressure in your wrist or finger.

Unfortunately, though they're easy to use, they don't offer an accurate reading. The American Heart Association doesn't recommend you use a device that measures blood pressure in your wrist or finger. Choose a device that measures blood pressure in your upper arm.

Additional monitoring tips

Learning to take a blood pressure reading correctly takes a little training and practice, but most monitors are generally easy to use. A variety of monitors are available at medical supply stores and many pharmacies.

Though many devices are available, not all of them have been tested to ensure they will give an accurate reading.

When you're choosing a blood pressure device, visit www.validateBP.org to see if the monitor you want to buy has been tested and validated for accuracy. Also check out the Additional Resources section in this book for resources that can help guide your selection.

For an accurate blood pressure reading, here are some additional tips:

- Don't measure your blood pressure right after you get up in the morning. Wait until after you've been up for at least an hour. Blood pressure varies throughout the day, and readings are often a little higher in the morning than they are later in the afternoon and early evening.
- Take a reading before you eat or wait at least 30 minutes after you eat, smoke or use caffeine or alcohol. Tobacco, caffeine and alcohol can temporarily increase your blood pressure. A meal, especially a large one, will decrease your blood pressure temporarily.
- Go to the bathroom before taking a reading. A full bladder will slightly increase your blood pressure.
- Your mood can affect your blood pressure. If you've had a difficult day, don't be alarmed if your blood pressure reflects that. Try and relax and take several deep breaths before taking your blood pressure.
- Check your blood pressure before you exercise, not afterward.

Benefits of home monitoring

Measuring your blood pressure at home is recommended for everyone with hypertension. Home monitoring helps you:

Track the progress of your treatment

Because high blood pressure has no symptoms, the only way for you to know if your treatment is working is to check your blood pressure regularly. Monitoring your blood pressure at home provides vital information between medical visits that you can share with your health care team.

Promote better control

Taking responsibility for measuring your blood pressure tends to motivate you in other areas of your program. It can give you added incentive to eat a better diet, increase your activity level and take your medication properly.

BLOOD PRESSURE READINGS — SAMPLE LOG

Date	Time	Systolic pressure	Diastolic pressure	Pulse	Medication changes/ comments

Identify usual blood pressure

For some people, going to a medical office causes blood pressure to temporarily rise to a high level (white coat hypertension). For others, the opposite happens — their blood pressure drops during medical appointments. Home monitoring can help identify or confirm your usual blood pressure.

Revisit Chapter 3 to read more about white coat hypertension and masked hypertension.

Save money

Home monitoring saves you the cost of seeing your health care team every time you need a blood pressure reading. This is

WILL I BE ABLE TO STOP TAKING BLOOD PRESSURE MEDICATION?

You've taken your medication faithfully, and your blood pressure is within a normal range again. Now you're wondering if one day you'll be able to stop using medication. The most likely answer is no.

Some people with high blood pressure that's well controlled can reduce how much medication they take daily. However, most people continue to take some medications for the rest of their lives. Blood pressure drugs ensure that your blood pressure stays at safe levels and can lower your risk of complications from uncontrolled hypertension — including stroke, heart attack, heart failure, kidney failure and dementia.

In a few cases, people with stage 1 hypertension who maintain a normal blood pressure for at least a year can discontinue their medications. But to do this, your health care team needs to set up a plan for gradually reducing the medication. You'll also need to see your health care team often to make sure your blood pressure doesn't increase again as you wean yourself from the drug.

To successfully manage blood pressure without medication, controlling your weight, staying active, eating well, avoiding tobacco and limiting alcohol are essential. Some people who successfully taper off blood pressure drugs eventually need to go back on medication.

If unpleasant side effects are the main reason you want to stop taking your medication, a better solution may be to work with your health care team to reduce or eliminate these side effects.

especially true when you first start taking medications or your dosage is adjusted. With these changes, frequent measurements help ensure better control.

SEE YOUR HEALTH CARE TEAM REGULARLY

It's vital that you see your health care team regularly to make sure you're getting your blood pressure under control and your treatment program is progressing with no serious side effects or complications. Regular follow-up with a health care professional is associated with better long-term control of blood pressure and fewer complications. Seeing your health care team every year is shown to make it more likely that you'll be better able to manage your blood pressure.

If you have stage 1 hypertension and no evidence of organ damage, your health care team likely will want to see you again within 1 to 2 months after you start a treatment program.

During that first follow-up visit, your health care team will look at your progress, see if your blood pressure has decreased, ask how efforts are going to change your lifestyle and check if you're having any medication side effects. If your blood pressure hasn't decreased, your health care team may adjust your program.

If you have stage 2 hypertension and other medical problems that complicate your treatment, you may need to see your health care team more often — maybe every 2 to 4 weeks until your blood pressure is under control.

Once your blood pressure is well controlled, a visit to your health care team once or twice a year is often all that's needed, unless you have a coexisting medical condition. Then, you'll need appointments more often.

Follow-up visits typically involve measuring your blood pressure at least twice, getting a general physical exam and having routine tests. The tests can show possible problems related to a medication or to a decline in your heart or kidney function related to high blood pressure.

Follow-up visits are also a good time to talk with your health care team about issues related to your weight, diet and activity level. These visits also give you a chance to review your medications with your health care team and talk about any side effects you're experiencing.

If your blood pressure doesn't match the target goal you've set with your health care team, you may be tempted to give up the program. But don't. Instead, talk to your health care team about why your treatment plan may not be working and consider adjustments you can make. Reaching a target goal may simply take more time. You can help by:

- Learning all you can about high blood pressure.
- Being optimistic and patient.
- Practicing good lifestyle habits, such as controlling your weight, eating well, being physically active, not smoking, limiting alcohol and managing stress.

- Reviewing all medications and supplements you're taking — prescription and over the counter.
- Seeking out a high blood pressure specialist if you and your health care team feel your treatment plan isn't helping.

Keep in mind that every drop in blood pressure from a higher level reduces your chance of health risks related to hypertension. Even if you have trouble reaching the original target, every step you take toward reaching it is one more step you're taking toward better health.

AVOID DRUG INTERACTIONS

The effectiveness of your medication depends in large part on you. When, how and with what you take your pills are important factors.

Taking medications correctly

You need to take your medications exactly as prescribed to get the best results. That may sound obvious, but by some estimates, only half the people taking blood pressure medications do so in correct doses at correct times.

If you take your pills too early, you increase the level of the drug in your bloodstream. This can produce side effects such as lightheadedness and nausea. If you take your pills too late or forget to take them, your blood pressure may increase as the drug levels decrease. And if you stop taking your pills entirely,

your blood pressure may rebound to levels that are higher than before your condition was diagnosed.

Know the names and doses of all the medications you take. Keep the original containers and periodically take them with you to your health care appointments to make sure you're taking the right drug in the proper dosage.

Here are some other helpful tips:

Use daily activities as reminders

If you take a morning medication, put the pills near your breakfast dishes, toothbrush or razor — so long as it doesn't endanger children or pets — or put a sticker near these items to remind you to take your pills.

Set an alarm

The alarm will remind you when it's time to take your medication.

Use a pillbox

If you take several drugs, buy a pillbox with compartments for each day of the week. Load the box once a week to keep track of the pills you take and when.

Take pills with water

Water helps dissolve the drug. If you generally take your pills with another

NUTRITIONAL AND HERBAL SUPPLEMENTS

Herbs and dietary supplements continue to be extremely popular, yet many lack sufficient research to fully evaluate their efficacy and safety. If you're taking a supplement — or considering using one — talk with your health care team about it.

Coenzyme Q10	Study results are inconclusive on whether it controls blood pressure.
Fish oil capsules containing omega-3 fatty acids	Many studies show that omega-3 fatty acids may help reduce blood pressure. Effects have generally been small, and other trials have reported no benefit.
Garlic	Evidence suggests it may reduce blood pressure slightly.
Ginkgo	No conclusive evidence it controls blood pressure.
Green tea	A few studies indicate a small but real effect in lowering blood pressure.
Magnesium and potassium	Some, but not all, clinical trials have demonstrated a positive effect with magnesium; more research is needed. More research is also needed on the effect potassium supplements may have on blood pressure beyond the potassium you get in your diet.
Vitamin C	No conclusive evidence it controls blood pressure.
Dark chocolate	Studies report a small decrease in blood pressure in people who eat dark chocolate regularly.

Supplements that can increase blood pressure

Ephedra (ephedrine)	Claims to promote weight loss, provide herbal high. Avoid. Banned by Food and Drug Administration. Similar compounds include bitter orange (Citrus aurantium).
Natural licorice	Claims to cure ulcers, coughs and colds. Avoid. Can increase blood pressure.
Yohimbine	Claims to increase sexual desire. Avoid. Can increase blood pressure.

liquid, check with your health care team or pharmacist to make sure it mixes well with the medication. For example, some medications should not be taken with grapefruit, grapefruit juice, Seville (sour) oranges or pomelos. (See page 126 for more information.)

Take your pills with food if recommended. Otherwise, the drug may not be absorbed properly into your bloodstream.

Ask for help from a loved one

Ask a family member or friend to remind you to take your pills, at least until you've made the habit part of your daily routine.

Use good lighting

Don't take your medication in the dark. You might unintentionally take the wrong pill or drop the pill and not realize it.

Note any side effects

Provide this information to your health care team at your next checkup. Your provider may adjust the dosage or have you try a different medication. Many blood pressure drugs can produce side effects. However, with the right medication, most people experience few problems.

Refill your prescriptions in advance

Plan to refill your prescription at least a couple of weeks ahead, in case the unexpected upsets your routine. Snowstorms, the flu and accidents are just a few examples of surprises that can delay your trip to the pharmacy.

Don't change your dosage

If your blood pressure increases even though you're taking your medication properly, don't increase the dosage on your own. Talk with your health care team first. Similarly, don't decrease your dosage without first consulting your health care team.

Consider combination pills

Many blood pressure medications come in once-daily preparations, and many combination tablets have two or even three different blood pressure medications in one pill. If you have a hard time following your medication regimen because you're on a medication that needs to be taken two or three times daily, ask your health care team if your medication plan can be adjusted. They may even help you spend less on your medication.

Preventing interactions

Many medications can be used to control high blood pressure. Some produce dangerous side effects if they're mixed with other prescription drugs, over-the-counter (OTC) medicines, nutritional and herbal supplements, illicit drugs and even some foods.

It's important to tell your health care team about all the medications you're taking and ask about any potentially harmful interactions.

Prescription drugs

Many prescription drugs can interfere with certain blood pressure medications. Some prescription drugs, such as hormonal birth control and some antidepressants, can affect your blood pressure level.

Many common anti-inflammatory drugs can interfere with at least four different classes of blood pressure medications: diuretics, beta blockers, angiotensin-converting enzyme (ACE) inhibitors and angiotensin II receptor blockers (ARBs).

Anti-inflammatory drugs counteract the effects of diuretics by causing your body to retain sodium and fluid. They counteract the effects of beta blockers by preventing the production of chemicals that relax blood vessels. And they reduce the ability of ACE inhibitors and ARBs to widen blood vessels.

If you're taking a prescription medication, your health care team can adjust the dose of your blood pressure medication to counteract any negative effects. Problems most often develop when you use anti-inflammatory medications here and there, so it's important to tell your health care team if you take such drugs, even occasionally.

Your blood pressure medication may be switched to something that's less affected by the prescription drug or your health care team may recommend or prescribe a different pain medication that won't interfere with your blood pressure medication.

Over-the-counter products

Pain relievers, decongestants and diet pills can pose problems if you're taking blood pressure medication. When taken with certain blood pressure medications, some of the following over-the-counter (OTC) products may raise your blood pressure.

OTC medications include nonsteroidal anti-inflammatory drugs (NSAIDs) such as ibuprofen (Advil, Motrin IB, others), naproxen sodium (Aleve) and high-dose aspirin. Low-dose aspirin (81 mg) doesn't affect blood pressure control. If you have hypertension, taking high doses of acetaminophen (Tylenol, others) daily is likely to raise your blood pressure.

Use cold and allergy products with care. Read labels to see if they contain a decongestant such as pseudoephedrine or phenylephrine (also used in nasal sprays). These compounds relieve congestion by narrowing blood vessels, minimizing blood flow to a localized area. This can increase blood pressure.

Food

Grapefruit, grapefruit juice, Seville (sour) oranges and pomelos (a form of grapefruit native to India) can interfere with the ability of the intestinal wall to process certain calcium channel blockers. This causes the drug to build up in the body, which can lead to harmful side effects.

If you take the drugs nisoldipine (Sular), felodipine (Plendil), nifedipine (Adalat CC, Procardia, others) or verapamil (Calan SR, Covera-HS, others), don't eat any of the citrus fruit mentioned above and don't drink grapefruit juice. Sweet oranges and tangerines generally don't interfere with drug absorption.

Natural licorice, the bittersweet ingredient often added to chewing tobacco and some cough drops, can increase blood pressure because it contains glycyrrhizic acid. This type of acid makes the kidneys retain sodium and fluid. If you take a diuretic to remove excess sodium and fluids, avoid natural licorice. Artificially flavored licorice — the kind often used in candy — isn't a problem.

Illicit drugs

Cocaine narrows and inflames blood vessels and interferes with the effects of blood pressure medications. Street drugs also can cause dangerous interactions. And marijuana can increase systolic blood pressure (the top number in a blood pressure reading).

Reducing medication costs

Many blood pressure medications can get expensive if you have to take one, two or three drugs every day for the rest of your life. Reduce costs with these tips.

Generic drugs

Once a pharmaceutical company's patent on a drug expires — usually after 20 years — other companies are free to

---

EMERGENCY WARNING SIGNS

In addition to dangerously high blood pressure readings, signs and symptoms that often signal a hypertensive emergency include:
• Severe headache, accompanied by confusion and blurred vision
• Severe chest pain
• Marked shortness of breath
• Nausea and vomiting
• Seizures
• Unresponsiveness

Don't drink or eat anything and, if you can, lie down until emergency help arrives or you get to a hospital.

make the drug from the same ingredients. This competition often spurs the original supplier to reduce the price. In addition, the cost of the new generic brands is usually lower because generic manufacturers don't have to recoup the costs of research and development.

If you switch from a brand-name drug to a generic form, don't be surprised if the new pills look different from the original. Generic drugs are often another shape and color. Because of this, read the label carefully to make sure the dosage is the same as it was for the original drug.

A generic drug doesn't face the same rigorous testing as a new brand-name drug. But the Food and Drug Administration does check to ensure that a generic drug delivers the same amount of active ingredient in the same amount of time as the original brand-name drug.

Generic drugs must meet the same standards of identity, quality and purity as required for brand-name products. Still, it's a good idea to monitor blood pressure more frequently when you first start taking a generic drug.

Splitting pills

Pills generally come in several strengths. Many times, higher-strength pills cost only a little more than lower-strength versions. For example, if your prescription is for 50-mg tablets, you can buy 100-mg tablets and split them to save money. You can purchase an inexpensive pill splitter at medical supply stores and some pharmacies. It's more convenient and accurate than using a knife and a cutting board.

However, not all pills can be split. For example, this technique doesn't work with capsules that have sustained-release granules. Nor should you split pills that are coated. In some cases, cutting negates the coating's effect.

In addition, the medication you take may not come in a larger dose that can be evenly divided. The pills must be cut into equal portions. If you're taking several medications or you have a condition that makes cutting difficult, pill splitting may become more of a hassle than help.

Check with your health care team or pharmacist before splitting pills to make sure it's safe to do so. If you do split pills, follow up with your health care team to make sure your medication is working.

Buying in bulk

If you have health insurance that includes coverage for prescription medications, it's important to know what your health plan covers.

For example, some plans offer reduced copays when you use a preferred pharmacy or a mail-order pharmacy. Also, quantities dispensed may depend on whether you're using a retail pharmacy or a mail-order pharmacy.

Comparison shopping for the best buy among pharmacies can be helpful if you do not have insurance coverage for prescription medications.

Discount mail-order pharmacies are another option. They can offer prescriptions at prices that are 10% to 35% lower than you'll find at some pharmacies. The discount is available because the clearinghouse buys and sells in bulk.

A disadvantage of buying in bulk is that if you stockpile too much of the medication, some of it may reach its expiration date before you can use it. Also, if your prescription changes, you may end up with medication you can't use. It's best to buy enough for only three to six months.

Another disadvantage to buying from mail-order suppliers is that you miss having a pharmacist who's familiar with your medical history and all the medications you're taking. But if you're good about keeping your health care team updated on your medications, discount suppliers may be able to provide a safe and wallet-friendly alternative.

Combination drugs

Some blood pressure medications are available as combinations of two or more medications. In some cases, but not all, the combination tablet may be less expensive than the cost of the separate medications in the combination. Whether you would save money with a combination tablet depends on the specific combination tablet and your prescription insurance plan. If the combination tablet is more expensive, you'll have to decide if the convenience of taking a single tablet rather than two or more separate pills is worth the extra cost.

Combination tablets are best considered after your blood pressure is stable and under control with the medications you're taking, and no further changes are anticipated.

If you take more than one blood pressure medication, ask your pharmacist if there's a combination pill available, and if there is, check your health insurance plan to see if it's covered. Then, talk with your health care team about prescribing a combination pill.

If you're concerned about the cost of your medications, ask your pharmacist whether a combination pill would save you money or if there are less-expensive alternatives.

Assistance programs

Some social service organizations and pharmaceutical companies offer free or reduced-price drugs to people facing financial hardship. Your health care team can refer you to the appropriate social services or drug manufacturer. Other resources that may be helpful in lowering prescription drug costs include Needy-Meds and GoodRx.

RECOGNIZE AN EMERGENCY

Uncontrolled high blood pressure can gradually erode your health by wearing down many of your body systems and damaging organs.

Sometimes, though, blood pressure can rise high enough to suddenly become life-threatening, requiring immediate care. This is a hypertensive emergency.

Hypertensive emergencies are rare. They happen when your blood pressure increases to a dangerously high level and are often accompanied by other serious symptoms.

Generally, a systolic reading of 180 millimeters of mercury (mm Hg) or higher or a diastolic reading of 120 mm Hg or higher is considered a dangerously high level. If you have another medical condition, lower elevations in your blood pressure also can trigger a hypertensive emergency. The danger level in children is lower, depending on their age and height.

A hypertensive emergency can occur for a variety of reasons. Causes may include:
- Forgetting to take your blood pressure medication
- Stroke
- Heart attack
- Heart failure
- Kidney failure
- Rupture of the aorta
- Interaction between medications
- Seizures during pregnancy (eclampsia)

To prevent damage to your organs during a hypertensive emergency, your blood pressure needs to be lowered immediately but in controlled stages. Lowering it too fast can interfere with blood flow, possibly resulting in too little blood to your heart, brain and other organs.

KEY POINTS

- Stress can increase blood pressure temporarily and complicate existing high blood pressure.
- Over time, the physical effects of stress can be damaging.
- Lifestyle changes, relaxation techniques and professional help can help you avoid or better manage stress and reduce health risks.
- Monitoring blood pressure at home helps you determine your usual blood pressure level, track the progress of your treatment and stay in control of your condition.
- If you take blood pressure medication, follow the instructions and take the medication at regular times.
- Keep your health care team informed of all medications and supplements you're taking. Many can interfere with some blood pressure medications or even increase your blood pressure.

Urgency vs. emergency

If at least two blood pressure measurements taken a few minutes apart produce a systolic reading of 180 mm Hg or higher or a diastolic reading of 120 mm Hg or higher — but you aren't experiencing any other signs and symptoms — contact your health care team if your blood pressure is still this high after you've relaxed for 30 to 60 minutes.

Most often, blood pressure rises like this when you forget to take your blood pressure medicine. If this is the case for you, take your medication and see if your blood pressure improves in 30 to 60 minutes. If your blood pressure doesn't improve in that time or you develop any of the emergency symptoms on page 175, go immediately to a hospital near you.

Left untreated for more than a few hours, blood pressure this high could possibly lead to a medical emergency.

EVERYDAY CHOICES FOR BETTER CONTROL

Many everyday habits, including managing stress, following the plan you set with your health care team and meeting regularly with your health care team to discuss your progress, are good steps toward treating high blood pressure.

Alongside eating well, exercising regularly, limiting alcohol and quitting smoking, these daily lifestyle habits can help you reach and maintain a healthy blood pressure level and live well with high blood pressure, preventing its effects.

Glossary

aldosterone. A hormone secreted by the adrenal glands that regulates the balance of sodium and water in your body.

alpha blocker. A blood pressure medication that blocks a hormone called norepinephrine from tightening muscles in the walls of small arteries. This reduces resistance to blood flow and lowers blood pressure.

angiotensin-converting enzyme (ACE) inhibitor. A medication that lowers blood pressure by disrupting the formation of angiotensin II.

angiotensin II. A substance that causes blood vessels to narrow and causes the release of aldosterone.

angiotensin II receptor blocker (ARB). A blood pressure medication that blocks the blood-vessel-tightening action of angiotensin II.

antihypertensives. A name for all the medications used to control high blood pressure.

aorta. The largest artery, which receives blood from the heart's left ventricle and supplies the other arteries in your circulatory system.

aortic valve. The valve between the left ventricle of the heart and aorta.

arrhythmia. Abnormal heartbeat.

arteriosclerosis. A condition in which the walls of arteries become hard and thick, sometimes interfering with the circulation of blood.

artery. A blood vessel that carries oxygenated blood from the heart to other tissues of the body.

atherosclerosis. A condition in which fatty deposits (plaque) accumulate in the interior lining of the arteries, resulting in narrowed pathways for blood to flow.

atria. The two upper chambers of the heart that receive blood from veins. Singular form is atrium.

autonomic nervous system. Part of the body's nervous system that controls involuntary actions, such as heart rate.

B

beta blocker. A drug that limits the activity of epinephrine and results in a slower heart rate and lower blood pressure.

blood pressure. The force involved in keeping blood circulating continuously through your body. Pressure is placed on the inner walls of the arteries by the pumping action of the heart.

bruit. A French word used to describe the sound of turbulent blood flow, heard when a stethoscope is placed over a narrowed artery.

C

calcium channel blocker. A drug that lowers blood pressure by disrupting the movement of calcium in the heart and blood vessels.

capillaries. Minute blood vessels that connect the smallest arteries to the smallest veins, forming intricate networks throughout the body.

cardiac. Relating to or situated near the heart.

cardiac cycle. The sequence of events that takes place in the heart from the beginning of one heartbeat to the beginning of the next.

cardiac output. The volume of blood that the heart pumps through the circulatory system in one minute.

cardiology. The study of the heart and its function in good health and with disease.

cardiomyopathy. A muscle disorder that makes it hard for the heart to pump blood.

cardiopulmonary. Relating to the heart and lungs.

cardiovascular. Relating to the heart and blood vessels.

cardiovascular system. The body system that provides a steady supply of oxygen-rich blood to cells and removes their waste. The system includes the heart, arteries, veins and the lymphatic system.

carotid arteries. The main arteries located in the neck that carry blood to the brain.

cholesterol. A lipid or fatlike substance found in the bloodstream and in body cells. People with high levels of cholesterol over a long period of time are at greater risk of heart disease.

circulatory system. Relating to the heart and blood vessels, and to the circulation of blood.

coronary. Relating to blood vessels of the heart.

coronary arteries. The arteries that supply blood to the heart.

coronary artery disease. The narrowing or blockage of one or more of the coronary arteries, resulting in decreased blood supply to the heart muscle.

D

diabetes. A chronic disease characterized by high levels of sugar (glucose) in the blood, often resulting in severe damage to the heart, blood vessels, kidneys and nerves.

diastole. A stage of the heart cycle in which the heart muscle relaxes, allowing blood to enter the ventricles (lower chambers) from the atria (upper chambers). From the ventricles, the blood will be pumped out of the heart and into the aorta.

diastolic pressure. The lowest blood pressure reached when the heart muscle relaxes. Listed as the second, or bottom, number in a blood pressure reading.

diuretic. A medication that increases the flow of urine out of the body. It's often used to treat conditions involving excess body fluids, such as high blood pressure and congestive heart failure.

E

edema. Swelling of body tissue due to the accumulation of excess fluid.

epinephrine. A naturally occurring hormone, also known as adrenaline, which helps prepare the body for danger or stress. It speeds up respiration and heart rate and increases blood pressure.

G

genetic. Relating to genes and to inheritance from parent to offspring.

glucose. A carbohydrate, also known as blood sugar, which is the body's main energy source.

H

HDL cholesterol. High-density lipoprotein cholesterol. Also known as "good" cholesterol. A type of blood cholesterol thought to help protect against the accumulation of fatty deposits in blood vessels.

heart attack. An interruption in blood flow to the heart, causing the death of a part of the heart muscle. Often caused by blockage of one or more coronary arteries.

heart failure. A condition in which the heart muscle is weakened and unable to pump enough blood to meet your body's needs.

heart rate. The number of contractions of the heart in one minute, which may vary according to how much oxygen you need.

heredity. The transmission of genetic traits from parent to offspring.

high blood pressure. A condition in which blood is pumped through the body under abnormally high pressure. Also commonly referred to as hypertension.

hyperkalemia. Higher-than-normal levels of potassium in your blood.

hypernatremia. Higher-than-normal levels of sodium in your blood.

hypertension. The medical term for high blood pressure.

hypokalemia. Lower-than-normal levels of potassium in your blood.

hyponatremia. Lower-than-normal levels of sodium in your blood.

hypotension. Low blood pressure.

I

inferior vena cava. A large vein from the lower body that returns blood to the heart.

J

jugular veins. Veins in the neck that carry blood from the brain and head to the heart.

L

LDL cholesterol. Low-density lipoprotein cholesterol. Also known as "bad" cholesterol. A type of blood cholesterol that, in excess amounts, tends to build up along artery walls, obstructing blood flow.

lipid. A fat or fatlike substance in the bloodstream and in body cells, such as cholesterol.

M

metabolic syndrome. A cluster of disorders of your body's metabolism, including high blood pressure, elevated blood sugar levels, excess weight and a combination of elevated triglycerides and a low level of HDL cholesterol.

mm Hg. An abbreviation for millimeters of mercury. Blood pressure is measured in these units.

myocardium. The muscular tissue layer in the wall of your heart.

N

noradrenaline. See norepinephrine.

norepinephrine. A hormone that's called into action when your body is under stress. This hormone increases heart rate and blood pressure and affects other body functions.

O

orthostatic hypotension. A significant drop in systolic blood pressure upon standing. May cause dizziness, lightheadedness or fainting.

P

parasympathetic nervous system. A component of the autonomic nervous system that slows heart rate, relaxes the gastrointestinal tract and increases gland activity.

plaque. Deposits of fat cells and other substances in the inner lining of blood vessels, resulting in narrowed, less flexible arteries and obstructed blood flow.

potassium. An essential mineral that helps control heart rhythm. It's also important to the nervous system and to muscle function.

preeclampsia. A condition that can occur in late pregnancy that's marked by high blood pressure and signs of damage to another organ system, often the kidneys.

pulmonary artery. A major blood vessel that carries oxygen-depleted blood from the heart to the lungs.

pulmonary veins. Several blood vessels that carry newly oxygenated blood from the lungs back to the heart.

pulse pressure. The difference between systolic blood pressure and diastolic blood pressure readings. A high pulse pressure may mean increased risk of cardiovascular disease and stroke.

R

renin inhibitor. A medication that reduces the production of angiotensin II, a chemical that causes blood vessels to constrict.

risk factors. Factors that increase your chances of developing a disease or condition.

S

sodium. A mineral that helps maintain the body's fluid balance.

sodium sensitivity. A response in certain individuals to their sodium intake, which can lead to higher blood pressure.

sphygmomanometer. A device used to measure systolic and diastolic blood pressure.

stethoscope. An instrument used for listening to sounds produced in the body, such as the sound of blood flowing through the arteries.

stroke. Damage to the brain caused by a disruption of blood flow, either from blockage of an artery or from a rupture in the artery wall.

superior vena cava. The large vein returning blood from the head and arms to the heart.

sympathetic nervous system. Part of the autonomic nervous system that increases heart rate, constricts blood vessels and reduces digestion.

systole. A stage of the heart cycle in which the heart muscle squeezes (contracts) to push blood out of the heart and into the aorta, followed by the diastole stage.

systolic pressure. The highest blood pressure produced by the contraction of the heart muscle during the systole stage. Listed as the first, or top, number in a blood pressure reading.

T

transient ischemic attack (TIA). A stroke-like event caused by temporary blockage of a blood vessel from something such as a blood clot. It differs from a stroke in that signs and symptoms generally disappear completely within 24 hours.

V

vascular. Relating to blood vessels.

vasodilator. A medication that widens (dilates) blood vessels.

vasopressor. A medication that increases blood pressure.

vein. A blood vessel that returns oxygen-depleted blood to the heart. Pressure in veins tends to be low.

venous. Relating to your veins.

ventricles. The two main pumping chambers of the heart, located below the atria. The left ventricle pumps oxygenated blood to the body, and the right ventricle pumps deoxygenated blood to the lungs.

Additional Resources

American College of Cardiology
www.acc.org

American Council on Exercise (physical activity tool)
www.acefitness.org/education-and-resources/lifestyle/tools-calculators/physical-activity-calorie-counter/

American Diabetes Association
www.diabetes.org

American Heart Association
www.heart.org

American Society of Hypertension
www.ash-us.org

American Stroke Association
www.stroke.org

dabl Educational Trust
http://dableducational.org

International Society of Hypertension
https://ish-world.com

Mayo Clinic
www.MayoClinic.org

Mayo Clinic Connect
https://connect.mayoclinic.org/group/heart-blood-vessel-conditions/

MyPlate
www.myplate.gov/myplate-plan/widget

National Heart, Lung, and Blood Institute
www.nhlbi.nih.gov

National Institute of Diabetes and Digestive and Kidney Diseases
www.niddk.nih.gov

National Kidney Foundation
www.kidney.org

US Blood Pressure Validated Device Listing
www.validateBP.org

World Hypertension League
www.worldhypertensionleague.org

Index

MAYO CLINIC | Mayo Clinic Press

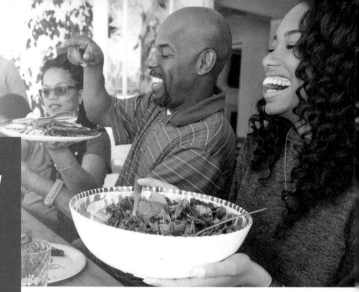

The Mayo Clinic Diet

Reshape your life with science-based habits

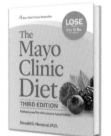

The Mayo Clinic Diet helps you break unhealthy habits that make you gain weight, replacing them with healthy habits that help you reach and maintain your target weight almost automatically. Unlike some diets, this is a one-time purchase — no clubs to join, dues to pay, or special foods and mixes to buy!

This sensible diet plan can help you prevent premature aging, reduce serious health risks like diabetes and heart disease, have more energy, and improve your quality of life

Just try the commonsense wisdom in **The Mayo Clinic Diet**, and we're sure this is the last diet you'll ever need. **Order your copy today!**

Cook Smart, Eat Well

Delicious recipes and easy strategies for healthier eating

Cook Smart, Eat Well is about eating better — and enjoying every bite. A healthy diet doesn't mean boring and bland!

Mayo Clinic Wellness Executive Chef Jennifer Welper creates delicious recipes that are tasty, enjoyable, and easy to prepare. She combines practical cooking tips with simple recipes that make healthy eating both pleasurable and satisfying.

In **Cook Smart, Eat Well**, you will find more than 100 original recipes with something for every meal of the day, including hearty comfort foods, savory lean meats and burgers, stir-fries, and delicious desserts. Chef Jennifer's methods will help you master basic techniques of food preparation, which you can implement with your other favorite meals.

Scan to learn more

Mayo Clinic Press publishes a full line of health books. Here is just a sample of our other titles:

- Alzheimer's Disease
- Back and Neck Health
- Digestive Health

- Family Health
- Hearing and Balance
- Home Remedies

- Osteoporosis
- Prostate Health
- And many more

Discover our full line of publications: MCPress.MayoClinic.org